NO LONGER PROPERTY OF
SEATTLE PUBLIC LIBRARY

WHAT TO
feed YOUR baby & toddler

WHAT TO feed YOUR baby & toddler

a month-by-month
GUIDE TO SUPPORT YOUR CHILD'S
HEALTH & DEVELOPMENT

NICOLE M. AVENA, PhD

WITH RECIPES BY CHARITY FERREIRA

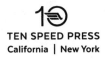

TEN SPEED PRESS
California | New York

Disclaimer: The information contained in this book is based on the experience and research of the author. It is not intended as a substitute for consulting with your physician or other health-care provider. Any attempt to diagnose and treat an illness should be done under the direction of a health-care professional. The publisher and author are not responsible for any adverse effects or consequences resulting from the use of any of the suggestions, preparations, or procedures discussed in this book.

Copyright © 2018 by Nicole M. Avena.
Front cover photograph copyright © 2018 by Ed Anderson.

All rights reserved.

Published in the United States by Ten Speed Press, an imprint of the Crown Publishing Group, a division of Penguin Random House LLC, New York.
www.crownpublishing.com
www.tenspeed.com

Ten Speed Press and the Ten Speed Press colophon are registered trademarks of Penguin Random House LLC.

Library of Congress Cataloging-in-Publication Data
Names: Avena, Nicole M., 1978- author.
Title: What to feed your baby and toddler : a month-by-month guide to
    support your child's health and development / Nicole M. Avena, PhD with
    recipes by Charity Ferreira.
Description: Berkeley : Ten Speed Press, 2018. | Includes bibliographical
    references and index.
Identifiers: LCCN 2018010055
Subjects: LCSH: Infants—Nutrition. | Toddlers—Nutrition. | Baby foods. |
    Child development. | BISAC: FAMILY & RELATIONSHIPS / Life Stages /
    Infants & Toddlers. | COOKING / Baby Food.
Classification: LCC RJ216 .A95 2018 | DDC 613.2083/2—dc23
LC record available at https://lccn.loc.gov/2018010055

Trade Paperback ISBN: 978-0-399-58023-9
eBook ISBN: 978-0-399-58024-6

Printed in the United States of America

Design by Lizzie Allen

10 9 8 7 6 5 4 3 2 1

First Edition

*"All grown-ups were once children . . .
but only few of them remember it."*
—Antoine de Saint-Exupéry

For my Prince, Star, and Sun
—Nicole

Contents

Acknowledgments

There are so many important people to acknowledge and thank for their role in making this book happen. Thanks to Sarah Veit; Katie Bishop, RD; Susan Murray; Alastair Tulloch; and Alyssa Emery for their editorial eyes and research assistance. I also would especially like to thank Kristen Criscitelli, RD, for her help with compiling the nutrient lists and advising me on foods to recommend, and Kristina Kunz Kharazmi for the information about Denmark. Thanks to my amazingly smart friends Suzanne D'Arcangelo, Julie Mennella, Alycia Halladay, and Alexis Conason for their expert contributions. I would also like to thank my wonderful editors at Ten Speed Press, Julie Bennett and Lisa Westmoreland, who have been a joy to work with now three times in a row! I would also like to thank the entire team at Ten Speed Press as well as Crown Publishing Group and Penguin Random House for their assistance and support in the development and production of this book, including my publicist, Natalie Mulford; designer, Lizzie Allen; production editor, Doug Ogan; and production associate, Dan Myers. Gratitude is extended to Charity Ferreira, who developed the delicious and easy-to-prepare recipes for this book. Thanks to my literary agent, Linda Konnor, for her wisdom, guidance, and honest feedback on this project and many others. This book would not have been possible without each of you!

I also thank my friends and family for their help and support along the way. I'd like to especially acknowledge all of my mommy and daddy friends, who have listened to me talk about this book, let me bounce ideas off of them, and allowed me to draw on their experiences feeding their own children. In particular, thanks to my lifelong friend Nicole Sette, who gave me such great feedback on early drafts, and special thanks to Clara and Faye Sette and Viv Blanchard for testing out some of these great recipes and food ideas. Thanks to my dear cousin Linda Hussey, for feeding my babies (literally) and helping keep things running smoothly at home while I was working on this book. I could not have done this (or much else) without you! I also am grateful for the support of my wonderful husband, Eamon, who unfailingly encourages me to do what I love. Thank you for keeping me going, knowing what I really want, and pushing me toward it. I also must acknowledge my dog, Bert. Thanks for keeping me company all those late nights and early mornings when I worked on writing this book. And finally, thanks to my two smart, beautiful, and loving daughters, Stella and Viv. You two little girls are the lights of my life and my best friends.

Introduction

Welcome to motherhood or fatherhood! If you're reading this book, you've most likely just started on the magical roller coaster of being a new parent. In between those nighttime feedings, endless diaper changes, and crying (with any luck, not too much!), I hope you have had time to take a step back and see how special you are. Being a parent is a blessing, and although at times it can be physically and mentally draining, it is the most important and rewarding job you will ever have.

Let me start off by giving you a little background on how this book came to be. As a neuroscientist with a focus on appetite and nutrition, I spend most of my days thinking about and testing how what we eat affects our brains and behaviors. I know that the foods we eat as adults can dramatically affect our health, and the same goes for a growing baby. I also have firsthand experience with the trials and tribulations of trying to eat well, both during pregnancy and when it comes to feeding a baby. When I first became pregnant with my older daughter, I was shocked to see how little nutritional information there was out there for pregnant women, aside from some guidelines about how much weight one "should" gain. That inspired me to write *What to Eat When You're Pregnant: A Week-by-Week Guide to Support Your Health and Your Baby's Development*.

When it came time to start feeding my daughter solids, again I noticed there wasn't a lot of helpful information out there in terms of which foods she *should* be eating. I knew from my research that there were extremely important developmental changes occurring in the brain during these precious months, and so I knew that this was a key time to support that development with proper nutrition.

I wanted to write this book to help new parents navigate the feeding of their infant and toddler. We already all know we are supposed to limit the candy and sweets and other unhealthful processed foods, so in this book I wanted to focus instead on how we can capitalize on all the *good* that foods can do to promote health at critical points during development. Also, I can tell you firsthand that feeding a baby well can be a challenge because babies don't always like to cooperate and things don't always go as planned when you are juggling lots of responsibilities (work, other kids, and so on). Since our modern food environment is rife with junk food and countless not-so-healthy, yet easy, choices, it can be tempting to turn to them (sometimes a little too often). So the goals of this book are to (1) offer guidance on what to feed your baby and toddler and (2) provide a plan for how you can actually do it!

As both a scientist and a mother of two little girls, I know one of the most important ways we can care for our babies is by feeding them the proper foods at each developmental stage. By giving proper nutrition, you can help your baby to not only stay well (we all know that there is nothing fun about a baby with a cold or virus!) but also develop taste preferences and food intake habits that they will carry with them throughout their life. You can make the most of when your baby eats by ensuring that each meal is packed with nutrients that are appropriate for each developmental stage and that you are choosing to offer them foods in a way that will encourage them to develop a preference for healthful eating. Yes, there is a way you can do this, and I will tell you!

Let Food Be Thy Medicine

Every parent wants to give their baby a healthy diet. But what does "eating healthy" even mean? All the conflicting information out there can make your head spin. Many parents wonder exactly what foods they should offer (or avoid offering) their little one to ensure their baby gets the best start. And parents want to know *why* this food is good or bad for them. The goal of this book is to give a real account of the science behind why what you feed your baby matters, as well as provide a practical plan of what to give them to ensure they are on the best path toward being healthy and developing a healthy palate. Your baby can grow up strong and well by eating foods rich in key nutrients at critical points throughout their early development.

How to Use This Book

There is a lot of information to cover, so I have broken the book into three parts. Part I covers *why* it's so important to feed your child certain foods at different points in his or her development. Chapter 1 discusses *why* eating good food is so important, especially in new babies whose brains are still developing and whose habits and preferences are still malleable. It provides science-based information about ways you can train baby's palate and develop healthful food preferences, the importance of textures, and how feeding your baby can help with fine motor skills and communication. In chapter 2, I focus on the basics of feeding baby, such as *when* you should start feeding her, how often you should feed her, and how much food she needs. In that chapter, I also cover many food-safety questions that parents ask when they start feeding their baby, including everything from GMOs to choking concerns. Since many of the tips and the information are helpful when you start feeding your baby solids, I suggest that you refer back to it while you are working your way through Part II.

In Part II, the real fun begins! I'll give you a month-by-month breakdown on not only what is happening with your growing baby but also what he needs nutritionally to have optimal health. Each month features a nutrient of the month, which is important for baby to get based on development occurring at that time. There is also a list of foods rich in that nutrient, as well as some delicious and easy-to-make recipes high in those important nutrients. In addition, I offer meal and snack ideas to help make feeding baby as easy and stress free as it can be. Following this month-by-month plan is a great way not only to optimize your baby's nutrition but also to test a variety of foods, flavors, and textures and get creative by trying some simple, fun recipes that your baby (and the whole family) can enjoy! In chapter 3, I explain the key nutrients that are essential for your child to have in these early days. That way, you can become familiar with these terms, as some of them are on the technical side. So it's okay if you have never heard of, say, manganese—I'll explain it, and, more important, I'll tell you why your baby needs it, how much of it he needs, and which foods you can feed him so he can get enough naturally. Chapter 4 focuses on ages 6 to 12 months, chapter 5 concentrates on ages 13 to 18 months, and chapter 6 covers the "big kids" (ages 19 to 24 months).

In Part III, I cover some more-specific situations and questions that may arise when you start to feed your baby solids. Feeding baby isn't always peaches and cream—no pun intended! As time goes on, sometimes it can be a challenge (or just darn frustrating) to get Junior to sit down and eat when he would rather be playing and surviving on milk and air. Chapter 7 focuses on how to handle eating in what can sometimes become sticky social situations, including eating out, day care, and playdates. Chapter 8 explores how to best approach picky eating as well as food allergies and other medical conditions.

In this introduction, I've touched on some of the unique challenges that new parents face when starting to feed their baby. In chapter 1, we will see in more detail why it is so important to ensure that baby gets exposed to the proper tastes early in life, and how this can impact her health now and later on.

PART I

Why the Right Food Matters

1

The Importance of Diet for Babies

Think back to all that you did to prepare for your baby during pregnancy. You probably bought cute new clothes to keep baby stylish and warm, and washed them in special laundry detergent to make sure they wouldn't irritate that new baby skin. You probably decorated a nursery and bought toys to stimulate baby's little growing brain. You also likely bought a car seat (and maybe even a family-size car—hello, minivan!), high chair, and other equipment to make sure baby is always safe and secure. I remember spending hours reading reviews and safety information on products to ensure that my babies were going to be safe and that I was making the best decisions about which items to use for them. When your baby was first born, you probably made sure everyone washed their hands before touching your infant, and you told people who were sick to stay far, far away. You sterilized bottles and pacifiers. You breastfed baby or diligently prepared formula bottles. You did all of this, and much more, to keep baby safe and healthy.

As parents, we have gladly taken, and will continue to take, all precautions to ensure that our child is safe and healthy. But what if I told you that most of us don't really give much thought to one of the most important things that we can do to keep baby healthy now and throughout their life—providing nutritious food?

When It's Time for Baby to Start Eating Solid Foods, What Should You Provide?

This might seem like a silly question to ponder. You feed babies baby food, right? It's fuel—calories they need to grow bigger. Well, science has revealed that it isn't quite that simple. First, we all know that our food landscape has changed dramatically over the past 100 years. We have become a society with foods that are genetically modified, doused with fertilizers and insecticides, and highly processed. These changes in our food environment have been blamed for causing not only some cancers and obesity, but also other childhood disorders, including attention-deficit/hyperactivity disorder (ADHD) and even autism (more on these topics in chapter 8).

Also, we have learned so much in recent years about how *what* we eat, especially at certain developmental periods in life, can not only influence behavior but also lead to lasting changes to the brain and body. New research exploring how food intake during early stages of life may impact a child's health and development has helped us to more seriously consider what we feed our babies in order to promote optimal health now and for the rest of their lives.

You Are What You Eat

Most of the recent headline-grabbing research on early-life nutrition has focused on obesity. In the past 30 years, childhood obesity in the United States has more than doubled in children and quadrupled in adolescents. The percentage of U.S. children aged 6 to 11 years who are obese increased from 7 percent in 1980 to nearly 18 percent in 2012. In 2012, more than one third of children and adolescents were overweight or obese. While lack of exercise has been implicated as one contributing factor in this outcome, the bigger culprit is diet. Studies show that, on average, kids (like adults) eat more processed foods than unprocessed foods, and processed foods are high in added fats and sugars. This lifestyle can lead to habits that are hard to break and food preferences that become engrained into adulthood.

Obesity later on is certainly a concern when thinking about what foods to offer your baby, but there are many other reasons why what babies eat is important for their health. Every week there seems to be breaking news about some food additive or ingredient that has been linked to the development of food poisoning, food allergies, diabetes, metabolic syndrome, and so on. Parents wonder, *Is this real or just media hype? Will my kid get cancer from the nitrates in the hot dog I fed him? Was there BPA in that can of soup I heated up for my toddler for lunch? Will my child be addicted to sugar because I bribed him with M&M's to sit on the potty?* These are just a handful of the anxiety-provoking questions that parents have about food—and that's not even considering the general challenge of just getting a baby to eat. This confusion in the media and lack of science-based advice was a major motivation for me to write this book. With mounting evidence of the need for good nutrition early in life, and with the questions and angst that can come with feeding an infant or toddler, it is essential that parents have a realistic, accessible, and hype-free resource to explain the new scientific findings in this area.

Also, feeding baby is supposed to be fun! So let's use new scientific information in a positive way. As science tells us more and more about infant and toddler development, we can apply what has been learned to support our growing baby's needs at each step along the way. You might have read or looked at other books that describe what is happening during each month of baby's life in terms of physical development and milestones, from rolling over to cruising along the furniture. We know that food is the best medicine and that many of the essential nutrients needed at the various stages of development can be obtained by eating a healthful diet. So in this book, in addition to discussing these remarkable developmental milestones that you can expect to see your baby achieve, I also describe the vitamins, minerals, and nutrients that can help support them in reaching these goals. But more on that in Part II.

Up until 6 months of age, babies typically live on breast milk or formula or a combination of both. (I say *typically*, as there are instances in which your pediatrician may have directed you to give baby water; for example, if he is severely constipated, the weather is very hot, or he has been sick.) But after the 6-month mark, he will need (and want!) to try new things. But what should you feed him? How much of it? In what order? So many questions may arise when it comes to feeding baby, and I hope to answer them all for you throughout the rest of this book. But first, let's take a step back to understand a bit more about what is happening with your baby developmentally, and why the foods that you choose to feed him in these beginning months can have life-long effects on not only his health but also his relationship with food.

FOOD FOR THOUGHT Breast milk or formula is still the main source of calories and nutrition for the entire first year of your baby's life. This means that what you feed your infant from 6 to 12 months of age can be focused on promoting healthful taste preferences and having fun learning to eat!

The First 1,000 Days

Over the past few decades, we have learned from science that what happens during the first 1,000 days of life (conception through the second year) can have a profound impact on health and well-being throughout the rest of the lifespan. As you will soon learn (or will know if you read my first book), key studies have shown that what a women eats while she's pregnant can have long-term effects on her child's food choices, body weight, and behaviors. We are also learning that what *the baby* eats early on can have long-term effects on her food preferences and behaviors. Yet pregnant women are given virtually no nutritional counseling, and most pediatricians don't delve into what you are feeding baby beyond mentioning the typical first foods to try ("peas and carrots, apples and pears" is the usual mantra) and perhaps, at your well-care visit, a quick lecture on food allergies and choking hazards.

I am hoping that the tide is turning, and—lucky for you!—you are among the vanguard of mothers who can take advantage of it. I am going to tell you what you need to know about feeding your baby the *right* foods, at the *right* times, to ensure she is getting exposed to all of the different nutrients, vitamins, and minerals that she needs to grow up healthy and strong, and with a taste for *real* food. And what I am going to tell you is based on science.

OVERDID IT?

If you are starting to worry because you ate ice cream every single day of your pregnancy, and Junior has been noshing all day long on those baby cheese puffs, *do not worry*! Some of the topics discussed in this chapter might seem a bit scary, but this isn't meant to frighten you. Rather, this chapter is meant to raise awareness about the science regarding the relationship between what we eat and a baby's development and to underscore why it is so important to consider what we are feeding baby. While some studies might suggest an elevated risk for certain conditions from a history of a poor diet, this doesn't mean these conditions *will definitely* develop. Also, by changing feeding habits now—with help from the food ideas in Part II and practical tips in Part III—you can get baby on the best path to health.

what to feed your baby & toddler

Baby Steps

During your baby's first 1,000 days, she changes dramatically, both physically and developmentally, from a pinhead-sized embryo to a walking, talking, dancing, hugging chunk of love. It's no wonder that science has shown us that the types of foods baby is exposed to through the placenta or eats after birth have a long-lasting effect: they can directly impact the development of the growing body, brain, and nervous system.

When baby is born, we see him as this seemingly helpless tiny creature, but one of the many things that makes our beautiful baby so amazing is the system of abilities and responses that he already possesses when he enters the world. We rarely give them credit, but newborns are a lot smarter than we think. Babies are born with cognitive skills, acquired in the womb, that lay the groundwork for future abilities and skill sets to develop; for example, baby can recognize your voice from hearing you while growing inside of you.

Famed developmental psychologist Dr. Jean Piaget called the time from birth through 2 years old the sensorimotor period. Within this time, your baby starts to explore the world by using her senses and actions to learn and grow, including the development of basic reflexes (such as sucking and grasping) and later, complex sensory and motor skills (such as walking and playing with toys). Your baby is essentially learning how her body can interact with her environment. This is why your baby will put *everything* in her mouth, including toys and even her own feet. This is how she explores and learns what each unfamiliar item is.

During the first half of the sensorimotor period (birth to 12 months), babies will come to repeat behaviors that are pleasurable to them. And during the second half (13 to 24 months), they begin to imitate others—probably, in part, because they derive reward from the interaction and fun of playing with the person they are imitating. This explains why they find peekaboo so darn funny!

And this has a *lot* to do with feeding your baby. By knowing two key biological facts—(1) that babies are programmed to be in an orally fixated stage and (2) that they repeat experiences that are pleasurable (and later come to mimic others for fun)—we can harness this information to help feed baby foods that we know she will like, and also model food-related behaviors when we know she will be copying them.

Negative Outcomes of Unhealthy Diet Early in Life

We have long known that what a woman is exposed to while she is pregnant can have a lasting effect on the growing baby. Babies who are exposed in the womb to addictive drugs like cocaine or heroin can be born addicted to these drugs. Not only that, children often suffer from long-term deficits in behavioral functioning (including difficulty with self-regulation), cognitive functioning, and information processing that all can be linked back to the damage caused by exposure to something in the womb.

But can exposure to foods have an equally strong effect? A classic example from history that relates early food intake to health later in life is the Dutch Winter Hunger. In 1944, there was a famine in parts of Europe, and access to food was limited for many people, including pregnant women. Studies that followed people over the course of this time and later in life discovered that the babies born to women who were exposed to the famine early in the pregnancy were more likely to be obese later in life. It was later proposed that by being exposed to conditions of hunger during a critical period of brain development early in a pregnancy, the babies were "wired" to adapt to hunger in order to survive. But later in life, when they weren't starving and food was abundant, they behaved as if they were still starving, thus becoming overweight or obese. This offers compelling evidence that, even over the course of a few short weeks, food intake patterns can have a long-term effect on a growing baby.

We also know that malnutrition (especially protein deficiency) in children is associated with cognitive or learning impairments. While malnutrition is typically associated with severe weight loss, that is not always the case. In the United States especially, many children are overweight but still malnourished. Malnourishment has pretty much nothing to do with calories; rather, it concerns the *nutrients* that one needs to remain healthy. The typical American diet is calorie rich, but nutrient poor. So many little kids look perfectly fine on the outside (perhaps in some cases with a little extra baby fat!), but on the inside, they are not.

You might find this surprising, but many children (and adults) in the United States are malnourished. Studies suggest that approximately 85 percent of Americans do not consume the Food and Drug Administration (FDA) recommended daily intakes of the most important nutrients necessary for proper physical and mental development. *More than half* of American kids do not get enough of vitamins D and E, and more than a quarter of them do not get enough calcium, magnesium, or vitamin A. Deficiencies in these nutrients have been linked to weakened immune systems, stunted physical growth, reduced mental ability, and chronic diseases. Scary stuff, right? But if you think your child might be a part of this group, don't worry. Changing one's diet now can begin reversing any damage that these deficiencies may have caused.

Several other studies have been done to better understand the role of the "food environment" early in life. Research in my own lab, for example, has shown that when lab rats overeat a junk-food diet (a high-fat and/or high-sugar diet) while pregnant, they give birth to baby rats that not only are prone to overeat and become overweight as adults but also are more sensitive to drugs of abuse, like alcohol or amphetamine.

How can a mother's eating too much junk food while pregnant lead to the child's drug use later on? It turns out that many of the same brain systems activated by eating highly processed foods that are overly sweet, salty, and high in fat are the same ones activated by drugs of abuse. That is a reason it feels so good to eat crunchy salty chips, sweet creamy ice cream, and/or sweet gooey cake, especially if you are having a bad day! Scientists have shown that overconsumption of junk food during pregnancy can actually program the fetal brain system in ways that may promote addiction. Now, this doesn't mean that you should toss out all the ice cream in your freezer once you get a positive pregnancy test. These studies suggest that *overconsumption* can produce these behaviors and brain changes but consumption in moderation does not have the same effect. The challenge is that it can be difficult to consume such foods in moderation, so many of us overeat and might not even realize it.

What do we know about babies' food exposure and health *after* they are born? The answer is, surprisingly, not as much as we should. The human brain is still developing until a person is approximately 25 years old (and even after that we know changes occur and new neurons can emerge). Compared to the number of studies that have been done on nutrition during adulthood, very few studies have looked at nutrition and postnatal development (up to age 5 years). Yet much like pregnancy, this early age is a critical window for brain development, especially for neural plasticity, cognitive development, and inhibitory control.

WHICH NUTRIENTS ARE WE LACKING?

Many American diets are lacking in common plant-derived nutrients, such as magnesium and vitamins C, E, and A. And more than half of Americans are running low on vitamin D. This is largely due to the fact that so much of our diet is now made up of processed foods, which are engineered to taste good but often lack the essential nutrients we need to remain in a healthy balance.

Early Establishment of Healthy Food Preferences

Okay, here is where the bad news stops!

We now know why too much unhealthy food early in life can be detrimental to health. But did you know that you can harness what we have learned from science to teach your kids to actually *prefer* to eat healthy food? I have the recipe for you right here (no pun intended!).

Studies of the relationship between food early in life and food preferences later on reveal that much of the action happens during pregnancy and while breastfeeding. Research shows that infants learn about the types of foods eaten by their mothers during pregnancy and lactation. These experiences of "tasting" the food via the placenta or through hints of it that come through breast milk have been shown to bias the child's acceptance of particular flavors and may even "program" later food preferences. This is one way in which culture-specific food preferences are likely initiated early in life.

In one classic study, food researcher Dr. Julie Mennella found that babies were more accepting of eating carrots (meaning they made fewer faces of disgust, mothers thought they liked the food, and baby actually ate more) if

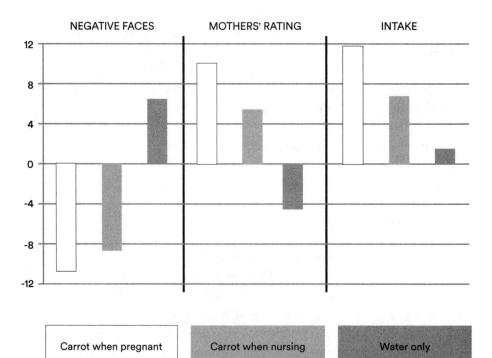

Source: Adapted from Mennella JA, Jagnow CP, and Beauchamp GK. (2001) Prenatal and postnatal flavor learning by human infants. *Pediatrics*; 107(6):E88.

what to feed your baby & toddler

their mothers had consumed carrots while pregnant or breastfeeding. And the amount of carrots that mothers needed to consume was not excessive. (It was a glass of carrot juice a day, four days per week, for a few weeks.) So if you are pregnant or nursing, this is even more of a reason to make sure you are eating (or drinking) your veggies!

But what if you've already had your baby, or you aren't nursing? The good news is that you can get similar effects on baby's acceptance of foods by starting her on the right path when you begin feeding. I'll explain how.

What to Feed Your Baby

Many of the illnesses that modern society is presently battling stem, in large part, from poor food choices. To promote health and, ideally, prevent disease, recent government guidelines recommend limiting consumption of salt, fat, and added sugars, and increasing consumption of fruits and vegetables. Not only are fruits and vegetables important sources of a wide range of vital micronutrients (covered in greater detail in chapter 3) but evidence also suggests that increased consumption of these foods can reduce the risks of chronic diseases, including cardiovascular diseases and certain cancers. Plus, eating more fruits and vegetables (and less of the not-so-healthy foods out there) can help both children and adults maintain a healthy body weight.

> **FOOD FOR THOUGHT** Despite the recommendations of health professionals worldwide, young children eat too much salt, fat, and sugars and too few fruits and vegetables; note that children tend to be more enthusiastic about and willing to eat fruits than vegetables.

While we all know that baby *should* eat more fruits and vegetables, in reality most aren't getting nearly enough. One in three infants aged 6 to about 8.5 months and one in five infants aged 9 to about 11.5 months does not consume *any* fruit or vegetable on a given day. Yes, you read that right. *Any*, as in *none*. Instead, young children are more likely consuming potatoes (most likely as french fries), sweet and salty snacks, and sugary drinks (like juices and soft drinks).

So, knowing the importance of fruits and vegetables, it is important to make these a staple in your baby's diet. But more important, it is essential to get baby to *like* them and to *want* to eat them later on when it comes time to feed himself and make his own food choices. How can you do that?

Repetition, Repetition, Repetition

Feeding a baby for the first time is fun and exciting, for all parties involved. Who doesn't love to see the video of a baby's face after trying a new food for the first time? However, amid all the excitement, parents often make one of *the biggest mistakes* they can when it comes to baby's diet and probably don't even realize it: they are trying too many different foods too quickly.

Research has shown that regardless of whether infants are breastfed, formula fed, or both, once they transition to solid foods, acceptance of fruits and vegetables increases most when the baby is *repeatedly* exposed to each one.

Most feeding guidelines don't follow this advice, though. Typically, they suggest trying rice or barley for a few days (you can actually skip giving grains altogether if you want; more on that on page 89) and then adding a fruit or veggie. Usually, 2 to 3 days of exposure is given before a new food is suggested to be introduced. While 2 to 3 days may be sufficient to alert you to the presence of an allergic reaction, studies show you need more time to establish *liking* of a food.

How much more time? Between 8 and 10 days. That might sound like a lifetime to you (and your baby), but that will give you the best chance of creating a strong preference for these foods (especially vegetables). Remember, when you feed a baby, she needs to actually taste the food in order to create an experience with it. Often, this feeding is messy, as baby spits it out or fusses at new tastes. Studies show that the more days a baby is exposed to a food, the more likely her facial expressions are to change to suggest she likes it, and the more likely moms are to report that they think the baby likes it.

EXPERT'S ADVICE: DR. JULIE MENNELLA ————————————

For the past 30 years, Dr. Julie Mennella has been studying the senses that define flavor. Her studies focus on how these senses function early in life and how infants learn before their first taste of solid food by experiencing flavors, transmitted from their mothers' diets, in the amniotic fluid and breast milk. What is her advice on how to get your baby to eat healthy? "Eat the healthy foods you enjoy while pregnant and then after the baby is born. And once your baby starts eating solid foods, he continues to learn. Tasting a variety of fruit or vegetables for 8 to 10 days increases baby's liking of these foods."

Sweetening the Pot

We know that our babies see the world very differently from how we do. With their brains still developing, they don't process emotions or restraint as adults do, nor can they understand concepts such as fairness (hence, the terrible twos!). It turns out that young children also live in a taste world that's very different from the adult one. Our brains have been biologically programmed such that early in life our sensory systems detect and prefer calorie- and mineral-rich foods that taste sweet or salty, while rejecting the potentially toxic ones that taste bitter (like cruciferous vegetables, such as broccoli). This is because in nature, sweet and salty foods tend to be safe to consume, while bitterness is often a sign that the food has gone bad (think about a fermented piece of fruit that may have fallen from a tree). So there is a biological basis to why kids like candy and don't like most veggies! Babies naturally prefer sweeter things more than adults do.

But we can capitalize on this. A clinical study found that school-aged children liked vegetables better if they were sweetened. So even though children have been biologically programmed to be leery of bitter foods, their preference for sweet and salt at a young age can actually trump the dislike of bitter tastes. For example, a study in babies showed that repeated exposure to green beans and/or peaches increased intake (as I said earlier, 8 to 10 days of exposure is best), but only the babies who ate the peaches *right after* green beans appeared to *like* the taste of the green beans more after the 8 days of exposure. It may be that the sweet taste of peaches masked some of the bitterness of the green beans, increasing their palatability and making it easier for the baby to like. When vegetables are given alone, studies show that it takes longer (more than 8 days) for the babies' facial expressions to indicate they actually like the food.

If you consume alcohol, think back to your first experiences with hard liquor. Did you ever do a shot of alcohol and then "chase it" with something better tasting right afterward? The same process applies here. The sweetness of fruit (or even a preferred vegetable) can mask the more challenging taste of the veggies. And the beauty of this is that baby comes to associate the vegetable with tasting good (just as you may somehow still have fond memories of that disgusting-tasting shot). If you do this type of pairing enough (veggies chased with fruit) with your baby, eventually you can phase out the fruit. This is classical psychological conditioning.

This has a few important implications for your baby's diet. First, if your child is really resistant to vegetables, you can try offering a fruit as the next mouthful. You can also try to use blends of vegetables and other ingredients to mask the bitterness. (More on this, along with some fun recipes to try, in Part II.)

Also, parents and caregivers should remember that "liking" and "intake" are not the same. You want baby to *like* the food, not just eat it. It is important to watch his facial expressions and use your intuition as to whether he is just swallowing what you spoon into his mouth or if he might actually be looking forward to the next bite. When a baby opens up wide, sticks his tongue out, and doesn't grimace or shudder at the taste, these are good signs that he is starting to prefer the flavor.

THE TRUTH ABOUT SUGAR

Sugar's reputation as a neutral (if not beneficial) food choice has been called into question lately, and rightfully so. Added-sugar consumption is on the rise, and it has been linked to many diseases and blamed for the obesity epidemic.

But is sugar from fruit also bad?

No, it's not—in its natural form, that is, and eaten in balance with other less-sweet foods. Fruits do contain sugar naturally, but in appropriate amounts and in balance with fiber and other nutrients that are beneficial to baby. However, be mindful that it can be easy for baby to start getting most of her calories from fruit sugar, and that isn't good (even if they are from fresh fruits) because we want baby to have a well-rounded diet. Many commercial baby-food blends are mostly fruits, with a few vegetables snuck in there. Remember, we want baby to get her vegetables and also develop a taste for them! So if you are giving food blends, try to slowly lessen the amount of fruit.

FOOD FOR THOUGHT You want to avoid any baby foods that use "fruit concentrate" or "fruit juice concentrate." Generally, the fruit is used this way to increase the sweetness. *Concentrate* is a sneaky way of saying that manufacturers have sucked out all of the fiber and most of the nutrition from the fruit, and all that remains is the sugar.

***

If you weren't convinced already, you now know why eating healthy, nutritious foods early in life is critical for baby. You also know that to boost baby's fruit and veggie intake, it's best to shoot for 8 days or more of exposure before trying something else. Next up, in chapter 2, I am going to give you all of the details, including when to start feeding baby, and how much he needs. Also, some great meal plans and ideas on how to introduce healthy foods to baby and get him to like them will follow in chapters 4 through 6. So grab your spoon, and let's go!

2

Feeding Baby 101: Do's & Don'ts

I hope that after reading the last chapter you are starting to feel more confident that feeding baby well isn't going to be as hard as you may have thought. In Part II, I'll be giving you a plan listing the nutrients your baby needs and the foods you can feed him to promote optimal health and wellness at the critical developmental milestones. But there is much more to it than just knowing which foods are high in certain nutrients. In this chapter, I will cover some of the basics for getting off to a good start: how much baby needs to eat, tricks for getting baby interested in eating, and some helpful tools to make mealtimes a bit more easy and fun.

IS BREAST STILL BEST?

The World Health Organization (WHO) recommends that you breastfeed your baby exclusively up until 6 months of age. So if you are doing that, great! But if not, that is great, too!

In the past few years, many hospitals have moved to what are being referred to as "baby friendly" environments. Long gone are the days when the baby went to a nursery so Mom could rest after many hours of labor. That baby is now bunking in with you! The idea is to encourage breastfeeding and bonding. And there is a lot of pressure on women to breastfeed, and a lot of judgment of those who do not. But there are many reasons why women don't (or can't) breastfeed. A fed and loved baby is best . . . *period*. Don't stress out if breastfeeding isn't working for you or if you are weaning baby when those first 6 months are up.

I will also address some common questions about food safety. One of our biggest concerns as parents is keeping our children safe. So it's natural that many of us have questions about food safety when we start feeding our baby, including everything from genetically modified organisms (GMOs) to choking concerns. It's an exciting time to get our children started on solid foods, but with so much happening in our ever-evolving food environment, you may worry whether you are making the best food choices for baby's health. In this chapter, I will try to put those worries to rest. While there are certainly safety issues to be aware of (which we will cover), there is also a lot of hype out there (for example, avoiding gluten without a diagnosed reason to do so). So we'll talk about what you need to know to keep baby's diet safe.

FOOD FOR THOUGHT There are some foods that you should *never* give to a small baby. See the table on page 37 for a list of foods that you should avoid feeding baby, and how to manage them as you do introduce them.

Getting Started with Serving Solids

Although the entirety of an infant's development is critical, the period between 6 and 12 months is a special time when you can expose your baby to a wide variety of tastes and textures, as discussed in chapter 1. By the time your baby reaches 6 months, the introduction of solids is ideal not only for her health but also because your baby is most accepting of new foods during the next 6 months. When you think about it developmentally, this makes sense: at this point your child is eager to explore and learn about the world around her. Exposure is how we learn to like new and different things, so why not take advantage of this opportunity to introduce baby to a wide variety of tastes, textures, and colors while she is most open to trying them? Early exposure to fruits, vegetables, whole grains, and other nutrient-dense foods has been linked to greater consumption of nutrient-dense foods and decreased incidence of obesity later in life. After 12 months, exposure to new foods seems to have less of an effect, whether or not your child likes the food. Simply trying to expose your child to new foods can become problematic, especially considering that between ages 2 and 5 years, children are particularly neophobic (meaning hesitant to try new things) about food.

FOOD FOR THOUGHT You may have heard you should avoid feeding home-prepared spinach, beets, green beans, squash, and carrots during early infancy, since these contain nitrates that can cause a type of anemia in infants. *Totally not true!* In regard to nitrates, the guidelines from the American Academy of Pediatrics explicitly say: "It is recommended that foods with naturally occurring nitrates (e.g., green beans, carrots, spinach, squash, beets) be avoided before three months of age." Um, *all* solid food should be avoided before 3 months of age! By 6 months, it's fine for baby to consume these veggies and others.

How Much Food Does Baby Need?

When it comes to babies (or adults, for that matter), I don't like to focus too much on calories or other numbers (like body weight, or servings per day) because eating a variety of healthy foods is more important than some arbitrary number. If you are feeding baby lots of different fruits, vegetables, grains, and proteins, and he is taking in food regularly at mealtimes, you don't need to worry about how much he is eating.

But it's helpful to have some gauge so you know roughly how much a typical baby at a given age needs. Also, it is helpful to have a breakdown of where calories should come from (as it can vary for infants versus toddlers).

Infants' (6 to 12 months old) total energy intake should be 35 to 50 calories per 1 pound of body weight per day. So if your 9-month-old baby weighs 18 pounds, she needs 630 to 900 calories a day from breast milk or formula and foods. To us, 630 to 900 calories might seem like a lot for a little baby. Most adults, who are much larger than babies, need 2,000 to 2,500 calories per day. Babies' needs are so high compared to their body weight because they are growing so fast, whereas adults need energy only for general maintenance (unless they are athletes or expending lots of energy each day; say, in manual labor).

ARE ALL CALORIES THE SAME?

Once in a while, a new finding comes out that turns the scientific field on its head. Recently, the age-old notion that "a calorie is a calorie" has been challenged. It is no longer believed that calories from all foods are created equal. An apple's 100 calories are *not* the same as the 100 calories from a handful of M&M's. So remember, nutrition trumps calories. You should focus on making sure baby is eating healthful foods rather than on how much he is eating.

When to Start Solids

You'll find a lot of conflicting advice out there about when your baby should be starting solids. By solids, I mean any food that is not water, breast milk, or formula. So that baby rice that your mother-in-law told you to put in your 3-month-old's bottle to help him sleep? Yes, that is a solid food. (See "Nap Time?" on the facing page for why adding rice to a bottle is considered a no-no). You'll find full details on introducing solids in chapter 4.

Before baby reaches the age of 6 months, all the calories, vitamins, and minerals he needs come from breast milk or formula alone. This means that there is no need to be giving rice, cereal, juice, and other foods before 6 months. In fact, if you do, you can actually cause problems for baby. Starting solids too early can lead to poor digestion, upset baby's delicate digestive system, or lead to uncomfortable gas and constipation. Because babies have an "open gut" through 6 months of age, whole proteins and pathogens can pass from the intestines directly into the baby's bloodstream. Babies start producing antibodies on their own at around 6 months, when gut closure also takes place.

IF YOU ARE BREASTFEEDING

Exclusively breastfeeding for the first 6 months decreases the risk of respiratory and gastrointestinal infection. Breast milk contains more than fifty immune factors and provides antibodies that reduce the likelihood of illness and allergic reactions before the gut closes; it also helps beneficial bacteria develop in the gut. In one study, infants who were breastfed exclusively for at least 6 months had fewer lower respiratory infections than babies who were not—and if the breastfed babies did get a lower respiratory infection, it cleared up faster. Another study found that babies who were breastfed exclusively for at least six months also suffered fewer ear and throat infections, and their immune systems were better protected for their entire first year of life.

IF YOU AREN'T BREASTFEEDING

You may be wondering whether you may as well start baby eating early, since much of the talk about waiting has to do with the protective effects of breast milk. But the advice to let baby's body physically mature enough to be ready to handle food applies to formula-fed babies too.

Nap Time?

Many new parents have heard that starting a baby on solids, such as rice cereal, will help her sleep longer and better. As much as exhausted new moms and dads want to believe this, there is no strong supporting evidence.

Let me guess—just when you started bragging about how good a sleeper your infant was, he started waking up at night. This is common and normal, and there are many reasons why a baby who has been sleeping through the night may start waking up—and waking *you* up—during the night. One reason is hunger, yes, but there may be other factors, like a change from familiar sleep associations (like falling asleep at your breast, or with a pacifier, or with the noise of the baby mobile over his crib) or sleep regression (this refers to normal changes in a baby's sleep patterns as he matures, entailing more light and deep sleep phases, with baby more easily aroused during the light phases). Sleep regression begins for some babies at around 4 months of age, and when that darling, sleep-predictable angel suddenly becomes a nighttime warrior, many parents want to try foods (or anything, for that matter) to get the baby to sleep again. But in these cases, hunger doesn't have anything to do with why your baby wakes up during the night.

It's also important to note that as babies grow, they need fewer and fewer nighttime feedings, as long as they get all their needed calories during the day. So if your baby is waking up frequently during the night, the problem most likely isn't hunger (or only hunger, if he is eating regularly throughout the daytime). Instead of starting your baby on solids earlier than 6 months in a desperate attempt to combat sleep problems, try to figure out the real cause and go from there. It could be itchy pajamas, noises from the heat coming on, or maybe even a cold, wet diaper. Put on your detective cap and see if you can figure it out. When my daughter started waking at night (well, 4:45 a.m. to be exact), we finally discovered it was because she could hear the neighbor's rooster cock-a-doodle-dooing!

You may have heard that offering your baby solid foods earlier than 6 months helps reduce the risk of developing diseases like celiac disease or type 1 diabetes, but as of this writing there is insufficient evidence to support this as a reason to introduce solids before age 6 months. The same goes for preventing allergies (with the exception of peanut allergy, which we cover in greater detail on page 188). You should always consult with your pediatrician if you have any concerns about possible food allergies in your baby; if any are confirmed, you'll want the advice of a doctor who specializes in pediatric allergies before introducing any new, possibly allergenic foods.

> **FOOD FOR THOUGHT** Many articles report that babies can start solid foods between 4 and 6 months. But you need to be careful about what you read on the internet! The major advisory organizations you can trust on infant health, including the American Academy of Pediatrics, UNICEF, and the World Health Organization, all suggest waiting until 6 months to begin solids.

Waiting the full 6 months allows your baby to become completely developmentally ready for the transition to solid foods. Starting a baby on solids too early is associated with increased body fat and weight when baby grows up. Research shows that every month a baby is breastfed in the first year of life decreases her likelihood of being obese not only as a baby but also as an adolescent and as an adult. Additionally, introducing iron-fortified foods (as you will read in later chapters, most baby cereal is iron fortified) too early reduces the baby's ability to absorb iron and can increase the risk of anemia. Some studies find that infants who are exclusively breastfed have higher iron levels than babies who start solids earlier than 6 months. These study results show that iron levels remain higher for the first full year of breastfed babies' lives. Breast milk includes a form of iron that is easier for babies to absorb, and won't irritate your baby's intestines in the same way that cow's milk can.

Finally, babies who start solids later can feed themselves more easily. At age 6 months, a baby can sit up on his own and pick up small items with his thumb and index finger. Also, the reflexes that babies are born with to help prevent choking gradually diminish around this age, which makes it more likely that your baby will swallow—rather than spit out—solid foods.

Baby Weight

Some parents may wonder whether a skinny baby should start solids earlier than 6 months. On the other end of the spectrum, they may question if they should wait past that recommendation before they start a chubby baby on solid foods. But the 6-month guideline is based on the maturity of the baby's digestive tract and the baby's developmental readiness, not the baby's weight.

First, if you have any concerns about your baby's size or weight, you should talk to your pediatrician. Babies vary *a lot* in size, so don't be alarmed if your baby is at the low or high end of the growth curve. The most important indicator of health is that she is gaining weight and growing each month. Some babies go at a slower pace at first and will catch up later on.

If your baby is on the smaller side, it's still important that you wait until 6 months to start solid foods. Research shows that for babies younger than 6 months, solid foods tend to *replace* breast milk or formula in the baby's diet, instead of adding to the total intake. Also, ounce for ounce, breast milk or formula provides the baby with more calories and more nutrients than most baby-safe solid foods, so it makes sense to stick with breastfeeding or formula feeding up until 6 months even if you have a smaller baby.

If there is one thing that many parents are sensitive about, it is weight (and I don't mean their own). Comments by others about baby being chubby, or skinny, are probably not intended to raise our concern, but they can have that effect anyway.

Parents can help a chubby baby by giving him healthy solid foods when he is ready at 6 months of age. Babies who gain weight fast in the first 6 months of life often gain weight more slowly after hitting the 6-month mark. So if your baby is chubby, you should still start him on solid foods at 6 months.

If you are worried about your baby's weight—whether you think she's over- or underweight—talk to your pediatrician. There is a huge range of "normal" baby weights. What matters most is that baby is gaining on an appropriate trajectory. Your pediatrician charts this each time you go for a well visit and sometimes will tell you the percentile that your baby's weight falls in. Don't worry if baby is in the 90th percentile for weight, or the 10th percentile. It is not critical, and odds are it will change by the next visit!

Remember, at this point baby is still relying on breast milk or formula for most of her nutrition. That is why you often hear about "complementary" food during this time. The food is meant to complement the calories and nutrition baby is still getting from breast milk or formula. You may hear a popular adage, "Food before [age] 1 is for fun." I agree with that but would add that it is for fun *and* for training baby to like healthy foods. So in these early months, you don't need to worry so much about how *much* baby is eating; focus on making food enjoyable and getting baby to try different foods.

IF YOU BREASTFEED ———————————————————————————

Breastfeeding mothers who want baby to continue nursing beyond 6 months have additional reason to delay solids until then. If you start baby on solids too early, he may start weaning before you are both ready. The more solid foods your baby eats, the less milk he takes from you, which leads to less milk production. If you want to delay pregnancy, breastfeeding longer also means that you are less likely to become pregnant for a longer period (although it is still possible, so don't rely on this as a birth-control method) because of the natural postpartum fertility disruption that happens when you are not menstruating due to breastfeeding. Research also shows that exclusively breastfeeding for 6 months will lead to more rapid postpartum weight loss.

When baby becomes a toddler, her calorie needs don't change all that much. Toddlers need to take in 35 to 40 calories per 1 pound of body weight per day.

Speaking of which, you might be wondering how *much* you should feed baby when you sit down to a meal and how often they should be eating. The American Academy of Pediatrics suggests that you feed your baby about 4 ounces of food at each meal (equal to about one small jar of baby food). While it is implied that baby has three meals per day, note that you can work up to this. When you first start feeding baby, it is fine to just have one or two "meals" each day for a few days, and those meals may be small (like 1 or 2 ounces of food). You can work your way up to three larger meals. There is no rush. By month 7 or 8, most babies are eating around 4 ounces per meal and three meals per day.

what to feed your baby & toddler

It is always a good idea to have a beverage (water) available for baby to sip at mealtime. Most parents transition from the baby bottle to a spill-proof sippy cup. However, that might not be the best idea. Suzanne D'Arcangelo, MA, CCC-SLP, a speech/language pathologist (and last but not least, mother of four) says that using a sippy may hinder your baby's oral-motor development. Drinking from a spouted cup, whether hard or soft, promotes the continued use of an infantile suckle-swallow pattern. As your baby matures, it is important to encourage the development of a more mature swallow pattern, where the tongue rises up to the alveolar ridge (the roof of the mouth) and sweeps back for swallowing more chunky textures. Use of a sippy cup may actually delay a child's feeding and speech/language development. Children with delays in the development of their oral-motor, feeding, and/or articulation skills may require speech/language therapy services to help support their developmental growth. What should you use instead of the sippy? The next transition from breast and/or bottle is to learn to drink from an open cup or a straw cup. This might mean more spills at first, but it's best for baby in the long run.

Snacks and Sweets: When and How Much?

The American Academy of Pediatrics suggests that when baby is around 9 months old you can start introducing two to three "snacks" per day. Don't let the term *snack* make you (or baby) think it needs to be a sweet treat or something unhealthy. A smaller portion of fruit or veggies can serve as a snack. Heck, leftover lunch can be a snack. If you can get baby trained early enough to see fruit or a slice of bread with nut butter as a snack, you can try to continue supporting this belief as she gets older and wants to have cookies and chips.

Snacks are a healthy part of your baby's diet. Snacking on healthy foods can help stabilize hunger and help baby learn more about food cues and how they make him feel. You might be wondering when you can start to add sweet treats, such as cookies, to baby's diet. Once baby is eating finger foods, he can certainly manage soft sweet treats, but many parents hold off giving processed food treats. I think it is best to delay these for as long as you can for these reasons: first, as mentioned in chapter 1, excess sugar intake has been linked to overeating and can cause addiction-like brain changes, and second, you won't always be able to determine what your child eats, so take advantage of this time in which you are still in control. Even if you don't make sweet treats a regular part of baby's diet, they will find their way in. Grandma will inevitably sneak your toddler a cookie, and baby will reach for cake at all those birthday parties and holidays, where you will have the added peer pressure to let him indulge (see chapter 7 for more on how to navigate social eating situations with your baby). Bottom line: If you want to give your baby sweet treats, make them just that—a special treat—rather than a daily habit (or a bribe or reward). If you can delay making them a part of his diet for as long as possible, that is ideal.

IS CITRUS SAFE FOR BABIES?

There is conflicting advice out there on citrus fruits, like oranges and tangerines, and whether they are okay to give to babies. While citrus fruits are very nutritious—for one thing, they're packed with vitamin C—they are also very acidic. This means that some babies, especially those younger than 12 months, don't have a mature enough digestive system to handle the acidity, and they may end up with terrible diaper rash (or even a rash around their mouth) as a result.

If you want your baby to have citrus, try it in small amounts, but be on the lookout for a reaction. If baby does develop a rash, it doesn't necessarily mean that he is allergic—you may need to just wait a while and try again. Also, be sure to either cut the citrus into very small pieces and make sure there are no stringy parts that could make baby gag, or puree it well.

Following is a general timeline for how much baby might be eating, and when. Note that this is just a guide, and every baby is going to differ. By no means should you worry if baby is not keen on following this plan, but it is a good reference for parents for the first two years.

what to feed your baby & toddler

Suggested Sizes of Meals and Snacks, with Some Examples

6 to 8 months

	SERVING SIZE	FREQUENCY/DAY
Breast milk or formula	24 to 32 ounces	On demand, 3 to 5 feedings/day
Dry infant cereal	1 to 2 tablespoons, mixed with formula or breast milk	1 to 3x/day
Fruits	2 to 3 tablespoons	1 to 3x/day
Protein-rich foods	1 to 2 tablespoons	1 to 3x/day
Vegetables	2 to 3 tablespoons	1 to 3x/day

9 to 12 months

	SERVING SIZE	FREQUENCY/DAY
Breast milk or formula	16 to 24 ounces	3 to 5 feedings/day
Dry infant cereal	2 to 4 tablespoons, mixed with formula or breast milk	2 to 3x/day
Fruits	2 to 4 tablespoons	2 to 3x/day
Protein-rich foods	1 to 4 tablespoons	1 to 3x/day
Vegetables	2 to 4 tablespoons	2 to 3x/day

(continued)

WHAT ABOUT JUICE? ————————————————————

According to the American Academy of Pediatrics, fruit juice should not be part of an infant's diet. If you still decide to give your baby fruit juice, hold off until he reaches 6 months of age and limit it to 8 ounces per day. Personally, I don't think there is any need for an infant or toddler (or big kids, for that matter) to consume fruit juice. It is mostly sugar, and water is a better choice.

Suggested Sizes of Meals and Snacks, with Some Examples (continued)

13 to 24 months

Your child's activity level, stage of growth, age, and appetite will affect overall portion size.* It is suggested that baby have three meals and two or three snacks a day.

DAIRY	2 OR 3 SERVINGS
Cheese	½ ounce
Milk	½ cup
Yogurt	½ cup

FRUITS	2 OR 3 SERVINGS
Cooked, frozen, canned	¼ cup
Fresh	½ piece

GRAINS	6 TO 11 SERVINGS
Bread	½ slice
Cooked cereal, rice, pasta	¼ cup
Dry cereal	½ cup
Crackers	2 to 3

PROTEIN-RICH FOODS	2 SERVINGS
Beans	¼ cup cooked
Eggs	½ egg
Meat, fish, chicken, tofu	1 ounce

VEGETABLES	2 OR 3 SERVINGS
Any	¼ cup cooked

*Based on recommendations from the American Academy of Pediatrics.

While it is a good idea to get baby used to mealtimes and a schedule, try to keep a flexible mindset. Baby will have days where he is not in a good mood, is gassy, or just doesn't want to eat at a given time. It is more important for mealtimes to be happy times than it is for baby to eat three square meals a day. So, especially in the beginning, focus more on the fun and ritual of eating.

Tips for Making Mealtime Fun

Mealtime should be fun for you and for baby. But let's face it, there are going to be some days when one (or both) of you just is not in the best mood, and then mealtime might feel like more of a chore than a joy. Here are a few things you can do to keep it enjoyable.

Get Some Fresh New Gear. Doesn't it feel better to work out at the gym if you have a cute outfit and nice new sneakers? It's motivating to get the job done when you feel like you have what you need. Same goes for feeding baby! Make baby feel special by getting him a fun new bib, a special meal toy, and maybe a cool placemat, plate, and utensils. And you can make cooking baby's food fun for *you* by getting yourself a baby-food blender (and see page 34 for some other specific tool suggestions) or a colorful cooler bag for when you and baby are on the go.

Let Go of the Mess. The mess will happen. If you like things clean and neat, you should make peace with the mess right now, rather than stressing about how much of a mess baby is making by dirtying multiple bowls and utensils, finger painting with her food (on the table, and her body) instead of eating it, and dumping her food on the floor. For now, your dog will take care of the big crumbs, and no one will notice the rest. Mess is best!

Change the Menu. Maybe you and baby need to change up the menu. If you have been feeding her commercial foods, try making your own! There are many easy and fun recipes in chapters 4 through 6. And baby would love to be your assistant chef! Hand her some plastic cups, bowls, and spoons and cook away together!

Go Out on a Lunch Date. Don't stayed cooped up at home. Get out there! Mix things up and head out to eat. I am a firm believer in bringing children to restaurants early in life. Not only will it give them a head start on how to behave in public but it can also help parents alleviate the sense of disconnect from the world that can sometimes develop when you are home with a new baby. If you are nervous about eating out with baby, start off at a family-friendly place where you get served relatively quickly and can make a quick exit if needed. Ask the server to bring you a to-go container when you order, just in case you need it. If baby fusses or starts to cry, don't throw in the towel and head home. Instead, head to the bathroom for a diaper change (if needed) and a quick change of atmosphere. See page 176 for more tips on eating out with baby.

GETTING STARTED: WHAT DO YOU NEED? ─────────

Here are some items I think are particularly helpful to have on hand when starting to feed baby.

Baby-food maker: To save time, opt for one that can steam and puree food all in the same bowl.

Bibs: You can't have too many of these. Opt for cloth ones that can double as a way to wipe baby's face. Also, I wouldn't spend too much money on these, as they are bound to become stained.

Cup with attached straw: When baby is ready to graduate from the breast/bottle, use this for offering water, breast milk, or formula.

Food storage: For storing extra homemade baby food, try small glass or plastic "cubes" with snap-on lids (great for freezer storage), or a good old-fashioned ice-cube tray. You can transfer frozen cubes to ziplock bags for storage.

Forks: When baby starts to be able to handle thicker foods and little bits, it is great to introduce the fork. I recommend first trying a few plastic options that baby can hold, and later graduating to metal ones with dull prongs.

Seating: You may need to feed baby in a recliner seat at first, but when he is ready for a high chair, I love the kind that doesn't have a tray and instead pulls right up to the table. It is a great way to make baby feel like a part of the dinner party when he has a seat at the table like everyone else!

Spoons: Have a variety on hand, as baby's needs will change as she gets older. Soft-tip infant spoons are for small babies; silicone spoons are for when baby starts holding the spoon herself. (They are also great for teething.) Also, have a baby-size metal spoon ready for your toddler.

Suction bowls: These can be useful for keeping food contained when baby is small (the bowl's suction base secures it onto the table), but I find older kids get frustrated when they can't move the bowl.

FOOD FOR THOUGHT After baby is used to the spoon, you can gradually increase the consistency of the food. If you are pureeing your own foods at home, you can thin them out to be the right consistency for baby by using breast milk, formula, or water.

What to Do When Baby's Not into Trying New Foods

Babies often balk at new tastes. They would rather stick to what they like (like your breast, or the ba-ba with milk). And sometimes we surrender the battle and give in. As long as they are getting enough calories, it's okay; right? Perhaps it is when they are just starting to eat, but not for long. Babies need variety in their diets, and they need to get that nutrition from food.

When baby refuses to try new things, simply keep offering! As discussed in chapter 1, it takes time and patience, but it will be worth it in the end. If you start introducing new foods and are persistent with it early on, baby will be less likely to resist when he is a toddler and has a *real* temper. Also, if you start good habits early and encourage variety, you will instill this in baby and help him go with the flow when you are in restaurants and away from home.

WHAT ABOUT PRUNE JUICE IF BABY IS CONSTIPATED?

You may have heard that prune juice is the gold-standard cure for baby constipation—but you also hear you shouldn't give her juice. So which is right? Many pediatricians suggest that it is okay to give a small amount of prune, apple, or pear juice if baby is backed up. However, I think you are better off giving pureed prunes, with some water to drink. Constipation can be alleviated with the combination of fiber and water. Baby needs the fiber and the water—period. If you give her prune juice, you aren't giving her fiber. The laxative properties of prune juice are actually from the sorbitol (a sugar alcohol) in the juice, not the fiber. But if you give her pureed whole prunes, she gets the fiber (and other nutrients that are sucked out in the juicing process) and skips the sugar rush!

Choking

The biggest safety concern associated with feeding that parents and all caregivers should be aware of is the risk of choking. While most people know that it is essential to keep things like small toys and tags out of baby's reach, choking on food is also a real concern to be aware of.

Each year, more than 5,000 people in the United States die from choking on food. Most are elderly, but it also happens to children and infants. If you have ever had the awful experience of watching a child choke on something, you know that it can be incredibly scary. It is important that you and other caregivers know how to react if baby chokes, and if he needs his airway cleared or needs CPR. Make sure that you and anyone else who cares for baby (including big brothers and sisters) take an infant lifesaving course. The American Heart Association sells kits to take the course at home on your own (see "American Heart Association" on page 196 or do an internet search on "Infant CPR Anytime Training Kits" for information on how to get one of these kits), so there is absolutely no reason not to be prepared!

You can avoid baby's choking on food by making sure she is developmentally ready to handle thicker purees, chunkier textures, and less-soft pieces. The tricky part is that there is no magic formula for knowing when baby is ready to move up. So you need to use your judgment and move slowly.

When baby first starts eating solids, the consistency should be thin. You want to get her used to the idea of opening her mouth and letting you put the food in. The first few times I fed my daughters, I actually used the trick of putting just baby formula on the spoon. That way, there isn't too much new going on at once, and baby recognizes the taste as something she likes and is used to. Think about it, if you put a new food-collecting bib on baby, and stick a spoon into her mouth for the first time, and it has some strange new taste on it (and there are gawking family members staring at her with cameras), it can't help but be intimidating. So keep it simple the first few times.

For ages 6 to 12 months, baby should be eating mostly purees, but as he gets closer to toddler age and starts to self-feed, those purees can include some small chunks. Just make sure that the chunks are very soft. Remember, baby can't chew his food. Those front teeth might look cute, but they really don't do much for eating. Babies this age "chew" with their gums, and by mashing food against the roof of the mouth. And even this type of "chewing" behavior doesn't come about until later on. Your 6-month-old will likely just swallow whatever you put in his mouth.

Foods That Can Cause Choking, and Measures to Make Them Safer

FOODS	WHAT CAN HAPPEN	HOW TO MINIMIZE THE RISK OF CHOKING
Chewing gum	Baby doesn't chew well enough.	Cut food into pieces no larger than ½ inch.
Chunks of meat or cheese	If swallowed whole, some foods can easily get stuck in the throat.	Supervise baby during mealtimes.
Hard, gooey, or sticky candy		Be especially cautious with round, hard foods.
Hot dog	Food stuck in the throat blocks oxygen from reaching the brain.	Have baby eat at the table.
Marshmallows		
Nuts and seeds		
Popcorn	If stuck in the throat for 4 minutes (or even less), brain damage or even death can occur.	Keep baby in an upright position.
Raisins		Make sure baby focuses just on eating.
Raw vegetables		
Thick peanut butter		Baby should eat only while seated, not while crawling or walking, or in the car.
Whole grapes and large blueberries		Have all caregivers of your baby take an infant CPR class.
		In an emergency, call 911.

Source: Adapted from Nationwide Children's Hospital.

Typically, choking becomes more of an issue when baby starts self-feeding finger foods. At this age (12 to 24 months), she starts to get more teeth, including those back teeth that can help her chew food. Sometimes this gives parents a false sense that baby can handle bigger bites, but she may not be quite ready—in part because she needs to be taught the appropriate amount of food to have in her mouth, when to swallow, and, if she is taking bites from a larger piece of food, an appropriate-size bite. While all of this might seem like second nature to us, some babies need more time than others to learn these basics.

YES, YOU CAN CUT A CHEERIO IN HALF

You can cut Cheerios into quarters if necessary. I know this because I did with my younger daughter. Every baby is different, and some have a more sensitive gag (or choking) reflex. For some babies who are just starting to eat small bits on their own, a whole Cheerio might be too much, so I advise starting by either softening a Cheerio with formula or breast milk, or cutting up Cheerios into smaller pieces. If baby seems okay with that, then you can try larger pieces, but don't rush. (Picking up those teeny-tiny pieces is great for developing hand-eye coordination.)

FOOD FOR THOUGHT In addition to the foods that are choking hazards, here is a list of five foods I suggest you should avoid when feeding baby and why, with more information beginning on page 44.

FOOD	WHY IS IT HARMFUL?
Honey (until 1 year old)	Can have bacteria that can cause infant botulism
Soda or bottled iced teas	High in caffeine and sugar
Yogurt drinks/fruit blends	High in added sugars
Too much cow's milk	Can lead to anemia and loss of nutrition from foods not eaten
Too much salt	Infants' kidneys can't handle too much added salt, and older kids get enough from salt used in food prep

I know this can sometimes be a challenge, but you should always try to sit with your baby/toddler when she is eating. It can be very tempting to put her in the high chair with her food and the TV on, so you can quickly to do things around the kitchen while she is an arm's length away, but by sitting together you will help her learn safe and appropriate eating behaviors. Also, just as you may have bonded with your baby while nursing or feeding her with a bottle, you can continue to strengthen that bond through your new role of nurturing her by providing delicious, nutritious foods. The dirty dishes, your work email, and social media checks will always be there, but you really get only a short window of time in life to sit with your baby and watch her eat, so enjoy it!

HOW TO TELL GAGGING FROM CHOKING

It's important to recognize gagging versus choking. Here's how to know the difference and how to minimize safety risks to your baby.

- *Gagging:* If your baby is gagging, he may push his tongue forward or out of his mouth, or do a retching movement to bring the food forward. Baby's eyes may water, and he may cough or vomit. The best way to solve this problem? Let your child continue to gag and cough until the food comes up.

- *Choking:* If your baby is choking, he won't be able to cry, cough, or gasp. You may hear him make odd noises or even no sound while opening his mouth. To dislodge the food blockage, you may need to do (baby-size) back blows.

FOOD FOR THOUGHT When your baby is very young, she has a tongue-thrust reflex that can cause her to gag or push out those first bites of solid food. Even after this reflex is gone, making your baby eat more than she wants or having too much food or food she dislikes in her mouth can cause her to gag. Some babies may even gag on their own fingers early on (my younger daughter used to do this all the time in her crib or in the car; it was terrible!), or gag on breast milk or formula. As horrible as it sounds, gagging is good because it helps bring food forward into your baby's mouth so she can chew it some more or try to swallow a smaller bite of food. In time, you will see your baby gag less as her body matures and she learns how much food to swallow at once.

COPING WITH CHOKING CONCERNS WITH TODDLERS ——

Toddlers think they rule the world. If they see older sister (or Mom or Dad) eating a slice of pizza, they want a slice of pizza, and they don't want it cut up like they are a baby! Ages 18 to 24 months is a time of budding independence, and while we don't want to dampen baby's enthusiasm for exploration, we do need to make sure baby stays safe.

As with purees, you should gradually increase the size of the bits of food you give your toddler, so that you can monitor how much he puts in his mouth. Also, don't put too much in front of him at once. My younger daughter was a bona fide chipmunk and would literally put the entire plateful of food that was in front of her into her mouth if we let her. You may need to enact portion control at first, so baby doesn't put too much in his mouth at one time.

When you (you, not baby) feel he is ready, you can experiment with giving him larger pieces of food to hold and chew off bites on his own. That way, you can monitor and teach him how much he should bite off. Always have a cup of water available when baby is eating and encourage him to take a sip of water between bites.

Organic versus Nonorganic Foods

We hear a lot about the dangers of pesticides and hormones in our food supply, leading many to opt for organic foods, which are supposed to be free of such things. But are they really any more nutritious or safer than nonorganic foods?

To meet the United States Department of Agriculture (USDA) standards, organic crops must be free from pesticides, GMOs (more on these shortly), synthetic fertilizers, irradiation, and sewage sludge. In raising organic live-stock, like chickens and cows, antibiotics or growth hormones are not used, and the animals are fed organic feed. Pesticides, such as persistent organic pollutants (POPs), are of particular concern because they can accumulate in our bodies due to their chemical makeup and overall resistance to degrada-tion. The main way in which humans are exposed to POPs in the environment is through our diet.

What are the long-term effects on babies exposed to POPs? Studies sug-gest that long-term exposure can be detrimental to humans. POPs have been linked to cancer development and neurological problems. Some types of POPs are also endocrine disrupters, which means they can mess with human hor-mones in ways that can effect baby's growth and development. POPs start accumulating in our bodies early in life, even *in utero*. And since they don't degrade easily, whatever baby picks up along the way he carries with him. The World Health Organization has stated that the potential health effects of POPs, especially among children, warrant global concern.

Hormone injections and antibiotics are often used in conventionally raised livestock to make the animals bigger (meat sells by the weight) and also keep sick animals alive (dead cows are worthless to a farmer). When livestock are slaughtered, all of the steroid hormones (or antibiotics) have not necessarily been metabolized, and some may remain in the muscles, fat, and other organs. This means, as with pesticides, when baby eats nonorganic meat he is ingesting trace amounts of those hormones and antibiotics. And studies have linked the use of hormones in livestock to certain cancers in humans, and also to the earlier onset of puberty that we are seeing these days compared to a generation or two ago. Even though the Food and Drug Administration says the amounts of hormones that remain in the animals are trace, that doesn't mean these traces can't affect our bodies. When a prepubescent girl is exposed to estrogen (even in small amounts via food), and she isn't yet producing it on her own, this can certainly have an effect on her health. More research is needed to better understand and tease apart the long-term implications of eating meats that have been treated with hormones and antibiotics.

So should you try to go 100 percent organic? Here is where I fall on this issue. Organic foods are not necessarily more nutritious for your baby, but they may be safer. Food companies can get away with using hormones, fertilizers, and antibiotics because the amounts that end up in the food that humans get in the grocery store are below the government-set thresholds. However, as I just mentioned, pesticides can build up over time in baby's body. And I don't think we yet know enough about the long-term effects of even small amounts of hormones and antibiotics that our little ones get in meat and dairy products.

TO GO ORGANIC, OR NOT TO GO ORGANIC? THAT IS THE QUESTION

When it comes to buying food, you should try to buy the organic versions of those that tend to contain the most pesticides (see page 42). There are also some fruits and vegetables that are "cleaner" by virtue of being conventionally grown with fewer pesticides, by being less likely to carry pesticide residue, or being enclosed by a tough rind or shell, so opting for the nonorganic version should be okay.

It is impossible to eat 100 percent organic. But some foods are more susceptible to retaining residue from fertilizers, so try to buy organic meats and thin-skinned fruits and vegetables. Also, diversify sources of protein and not rely on meats and dairy so much (see page 61 for some nonmeat proteins that are baby friendly). You can't totally protect baby from the harmful chemicals in our environment but you can minimize exposure.

Top 10 Cleaner and Dirtier Foods

CLEANER	DIRTIER
Sweet corn*	Strawberry
Avocado	Spinach
Pineapple	Nectarine
Cabbage	Apple
Onion	Peach
Sweet peas, frozen	Pear
Papaya*	Cherry
Asparagus	Grape
Mango	Celery
Eggplant	Tomato

*In the United States, a small amount is produced using genetically modified seeds.

Source: Adapted from Environmental Working Group's *2017 Shopper's Guide to Pesticides in Produce*

WHAT ABOUT COMMERCIALLY AVAILABLE BABY FOOD? — Many store-bought organic baby foods are available. To be labeled "organic," it must meet standards set by the USDA National Organic Program, including it must be made from fruits and vegetables that haven't been sprayed with chemical pesticides, meat must be from animals that haven't been given antibiotics or growth hormones, and it must not contain any artificial flavors, colors, or preservatives.

Generally, the price difference is not as dramatic as it can be between organic and nonorganic produce or meats, so if you are keen on organic baby food but are on a budget, you can still make it work by buying it commercially.

FOOD FOR THOUGHT Want a tip for when you're at the grocery store? Make sure to check the ingredient list on baby-food jars, as many manufacturers will replace real food with water and flour to thicken the consistency. This means that your baby will get fewer nutrients per ounce than with single-ingredient baby food.

GMOs

Thanks to the media, we hear a lot about the horrors of GMOs, but what exactly are they, and should you care if the food you feed your baby contains them?

Genetically modified organisms, or GMOs, are created by changing the traits in the DNA of plants and animals to achieve some desired attribute. For instance, a corn plant can have a gene added to make it more nutritious or more tolerant or resistant to factors such as weather, herbicides, or disease. Scientists actually have a "gene gun" that they use to shoot the desired gene directly into the new plant cell in the lab. In some ways, it is sort of like designer dog breeding (labradoodle, anyone?); you can purposefully increase the desired qualities (such as a certain nutrient in food, or playfulness with kids in a dog) and decrease the undesired traits (such as being sensitive to fungi in food, or shedding in your pooch).

In countries like the United States, most people don't need to worry much about the nutritional content of individual food items, as most of us have access to a wide variety of foods that can meet all of our nutritional needs. But in poorer countries this is often not the case, and people may rely on a single food crop for most of their calories and nutrition. So if there is a drought one season or the crop gets a fungus, people may starve. GMO technology is a way that scientists can alleviate some of these problems by engineering plants to be resistant to disease and environmental threats, as well as express additional features that can combat malnutrition.

Whether or not GMOs can be harmful to your child is a tricky question. Many people believe that "natural" is better, because when we play with our food technologically, human health and the environment can be impacted. While this is a valid theory, it is still just a theory.

In the United States, many regulatory bodies—including the FDA, the United States Environmental Protection Agency (EPA), and the USDA's Animal and Plant Health Inspection Service (APHIS)—are involved in GMO crop approval. Genetically modified (GM) plants have to undergo extensive safety testing prior to finding their way into the grocery store.

Here is what the data says about the safety of GMOs. Food from genetically modified crops has been consumed by hundreds of millions of people throughout the world for more than 15 years, with no known reported ill effects. There is little evidence that GM crops are toxic. One study suggested that rats fed GM potatoes had damage to their guts as a result, but this study has not been replicated and the findings have not been widely accepted among the scientific community.

Some are also concerned that feeding your baby foods containing GMOs might introduce new allergens and may lead to allergic reactions in your child. Testing for these allergens is difficult, experts say. However, GM technology might also be used to decrease the levels of allergens present in plants by reducing expression levels of the relevant genes. For example, research has been used to identify an allergen in soybeans and remove it using GM technology.

Bottom line: GMOs, globally, do a lot more known good than potential harm. But they also are still relatively new, and more research is needed to understand the effects of GMOs in our foods. I see no reason based on the current science to avoid them, but doing so won't hurt. Note that unless you buy organic (which must not contain GMO ingredients) it is pretty much impossible to completely avoid them, as most nonorganic processed foods (ranging from Twinkies to something simple, such as peanut butter) contain GM ingredients.

HOW YOU CAN REDUCE GMO INTAKE —————————————

If you are concerned about GMOs, you can do the following:

- Buy organic foods (organic foods certified by the USDA do not contain GMOs).
- Look for foods with a non-GMO label.
- Avoid or limit foods that are likely to contain GMOs (corn or soy flour, canola and cottonseed oil, and beet sugar).
- Feed your baby fresh fruits and vegetables (but note that zucchini, papaya, and sweet corn may be genetically modified).

When to Introduce Dairy and Eggs

Dairy can come in many forms, from cow's milk to butter to cheese to yogurt. Since dairy products as a class are pretty diverse, you may be wondering when it is okay to introduce each of the different ones.

Cow's Milk. Baby should not have cow's milk until she is 12 months old. If she is weaned from breast milk or baby formula sooner, cow's milk is *not* the replacement. Baby then needs to get her nutrition mostly from food, and cow's milk is a *supplement*. If baby has become accustomed to being fed with a bottle of breast milk or formula, there can be a psychological attachment to the bottle, and you may find that baby demands a "ba-ba" quite often throughout the day. So be mindful that baby may be filling up on milk and less likely to want to eat real food if you give in to ba-ba requests throughout the day.

CAN BABY DRINK ALMOND MILK OR SOY MILK?

Many babies who are allergic to cow's milk can drink soy or almond milk instead. But just as with cow's milk, it needs to be in moderation. And watch out for the sugar content. Many almond and soy milks have a lot of added sugar. Also, opt for brands that are also fortified with calcium.

How much cow's milk should baby be drinking? According to the American Academy of Pediatrics, a 12-month-old needs 1 to 1½ cups of milk (or equivalent dairy products) a day to get enough vitamin D and calcium. By age 2, your baby should get 2 cups of milk (or equivalent dairy products) each day. Remember, the purpose of the milk isn't for the calories but rather for the vitamin D and calcium.

MILK ADDICT?

If your baby (and you) have developed a milk habit, don't worry. Here are some things you can do to break it:

- Try offering milk only a few times each day, and the rest of the day give him water. If you give him milk in the morning when he wakes up, and then milk again before bed (making sure to brush his teeth afterward, as the sugar in the milk can lead to cavity formation), this can limit his intake.

- If you think the milk habit is really an attachment to the bottle, it might be a sign baby should give up the ba-ba and move on to a cup. You might have to deal with a few tears, but baby will get over it before you know it.

- Don't offer milk until after baby has had his meal. If you offer him water, he may balk, but if he is truly thirsty he will drink it and then eat food when he is hungry.

Butter. You can use butter in foods you offer to baby after age 6 months. It can be a good source of fat and can help promote the healthy development of baby's brain. Butter can be a great way to increase the palatability of foods that baby might not love, like vegetables. To change things up, you can use a bit of butter instead of fruit in your purees to help mask the taste of vegetables.

Cheese. You can offer cheese once baby is 8 to 10 months old, as long as she doesn't have milk allergies. (If she does, talk to your pediatrician about when it is best to introduce it.) Small pieces of soft, milder-tasting cheeses, like mild cheddar or Colby, are good to try at first. Shredded cheeses are an option too, especially for self-feeders. Cottage cheese can be good to try because it is soft, but avoid the kinds with fruit mixed in—these are usually loaded with added sugars. Avoid hard cheeses altogether and also be careful of melted cheeses, such as mozzarella, which can be stringy and pose a choking hazard.

Yogurt. You can offer yogurt starting at 8 months. Some experts say earlier, but I think that it is best to spend those first 2 months trying to get baby used to fruits and vegetables. Starting earlier than 8 months won't hurt; it's really a matter of your preferences. Opt for whole-milk yogurt, as baby needs the fat. But avoid yogurt drinks or yogurts with fruit added, as these are loaded with added sugars. Baby likes just plain ol' yogurt! See page 102 for more information on which types of yogurt you can offer your baby.

WHAT PERCENT-FAT MILK SHOULD BABY GET? ——————

From age 1 year to around 2 years, babies should be given whole milk. By age 2, you should be able to switch to 2% or 1% milk; however, if baby is getting enough good fats from other sources, you can switch earlier. People wonder if you should give a baby skim milk. Unless there is a medical reason that concerns you or your pediatrician, stick with the low-fat options. The fat in milk is healthier than fats baby gets from other sources as he gets older. People might think it's okay to give skim milk more often throughout the day because it is lower in calories and fat, and thus won't interfere with baby's intake of food, but this is not a good idea. You need to avoid overdoing milk (with any fat content) because too much can induce anemia in baby, as it inhibits iron absorption. If baby is milk-seeking after he has had enough for the day, you can add a bit of water to milk to increase the volume and make it last longer. I used this trick on my older daughter to break her milk habit, and it worked like a charm!

Eggs. Eggs are a great first finger food and good to offer baby starting at about 8 months (but if egg allergies run in your family, see page 185). They are loaded with nutrients and are easy to prepare and store. You can hard-boil an egg and chop it into small pieces, or prepare scrambled eggs, and let baby enjoy.

WHY WAIT FOR MILK BUT NOT OTHER DAIRY?

You can offer baby cheese and yogurt earlier than cow's milk for two main reasons:

- Lactose (the sugar in dairy) is already broken down through the culturing of the cheese or yogurt, and the milk proteins are either removed or very reduced, making cheeses and yogurts easier for baby to digest.

- There is some concern in the medical community that if parents are told they can give baby cow's milk earlier than 12 months, they will cut back on breast milk or formula, which baby really needs to get all of the nutrition these deliver. It is really best to wait until 12 months of age for cow's milk, so that baby's digestive system is ready to handle it, and so that baby is ready to get the bulk of her nutrition from solids (as opposed to breast milk or formula).

Oh, Honey!

Babies under age 1 year should *not* have honey (or corn syrup). Honey and corn syrup can contain spores of bacteria that can grow in a baby's immature digestive system and cause infant botulism (yikes!). Although it is very rare, it can be a potentially fatal illness, so it is best to avoid honey or any products that use honey as an ingredient (even if baked) until baby is 1 year old.

What about Salt?

Adults are well aware that they should minimize their salt intake to avoid cardiovascular problems and hypertension. Most of us get more than enough salt without even sprinkling it on our meals because processed foods are incredibly oversalted.

But salt (sodium) is a necessary part of our diets. Babies need salt too, but up to age 12 months they are getting what they need from breast milk or formula. Babies need less than 1 gram of salt per day, and their little kidneys can't process any more than that.

After 12 months, you can still hold off on the salt shaker. As baby starts to eat more finger foods and foods that the family would eat, he will likely get more than enough salt (and now he can excrete the extra, thanks to his matured kidneys). So if you add a pinch of salt to a dish you prepared and plan to share with baby, no problem. Just don't get into the habit of sprinkling salt from a shaker onto baby's food on the plate. Remember, for your toddler it's monkey-see-monkey-do, so if you add on the salt, baby will likely want a shake, too. Best for all to leave the salt shaker next to the stove to be used when cooking, not eating.

FOOD FOR THOUGHT Think twice before feeding your baby too many foods that are made for adults (like canned veggies). These can contain a lot of salt, in addition to preservatives, artificial colors, flavors, and other chemicals. Check the nutrition information on the label for sodium content, and look for "no salt added" and "reduced sodium" choices.

Gluten

Gluten is the protein found in wheat, rye, and barley. It is sort of like a glue that holds some foods together (making "glu"-ten an appropriate name!). Gluten gives dough its elasticity and helps to make some foods chewy.

These days it seems that every processed food comes in a gluten-free variety. Great, right? Well, sort of. People who have celiac disease can't process gluten in food, so they get very sick if they consume it. This is an autoimmune disease, which means that when people with celiac eat gluten, their body attacks itself, which causes damage to the intestines and can lead to issues related to nutrient absorption. Celiac is a serious disease; if left untreated it can lead to anemia, osteoporosis, infertility, central and peripheral nervous-system disorders, and gall bladder malfunction, among other things. There is a blood test used to diagnose celiac disease, and people who test positive need to be on a strict gluten-free diet. Celiac affects approximately 1 percent of the population.

FOOD FOR THOUGHT Babies can be exposed to gluten via breast milk if the mother's diet contains gluten.

Also, we are now learning that some people are *gluten-sensitive*; this means they aren't full-blown allergic to gluten but when their diet includes gluten they experience some symptoms found in celiac disease, such as "foggy mind," ADHD-like behavior, depression, bloating, abdominal pain, diarrhea, headaches, constipation, bone or joint pain, and chronic fatigue. However, although these people do not test positive for celiac disease, removing gluten from the diet resolves their symptoms. The terms "non-celiac gluten sensitivity" (NCGS) and "non-celiac wheat sensitivity" (NCWS) are generally used to refer to this condition. Because there are no biomarkers for NCGS or NCWS, it is hard to pinpoint the actual number of people who have it, but it is estimated to affect about 1 percent of the population (about the same prevalence as celiac disease).

HOW CAN YOU TELL IF YOUR BABY HAS TROUBLE WITH GLUTEN?

Babies are often little mysteries. They give us some clues about what is bothering them, and it is up to us to be the detectives and get to the bottom of it. Gluten sensitivity or celiac disease can be difficult to pinpoint, as the symptoms vary and are often associated with other health issues. Symptoms can include vomiting, gas, constipation, hives, or diarrhea. So if you start noticing these things, and you suspect that it is associated with food, talk to your pediatrician. She can easily rule out celiac disease with a blood test and then guide you in determining whether baby might have NCGS or NCWS. This is usually done via an elimination diet for 2 weeks to see if the symptoms resolve, followed by a reintroduction phase to see if they return.

So without knowing how your baby might react to gluten, and considering there are so many gluten-free options out there, you might be wondering if baby should go gluten-free? The short answer is no. Experts advise against going gluten-free unless there is a medical reason for it. In fact, it can be unhealthy to avoid gluten. Cutting out gluten can mean that your child could miss out on essential nutrients, minerals, and fiber. And although lately there is a lot more awareness about gluten-free diets, you may also find that eliminating gluten from your baby's diet can make food preparation (for everything from day care to playdates) more complicated and expensive. So if you are considering going gluten-free because baby has shown signs of gluten intolerance or gluten sensitivity, talk with your doctor about whether it's truly necessary. The key takeaway? Be sure that it's essential for your baby to avoid gluten before making any drastic changes to her diet.

WHAT ABOUT THOSE PEARLY WHITES?

Fluoride is essential for healthy teeth to prevent tooth decay during an individual's lifetime. Since baby teeth start coming in at 6 or 7 months, it's important to pay attention to the amount of fluoride baby is exposed to. Human milk is very low in fluoride, after tooth eruption it is recommended you offer fluoridated water several times per day to breastfed infants or that you prepare formula with fluoridated water. Be cautious—fluoride may be essential to prevent tooth decay, but excessive exposure can cause dental fluorosis, in which the enamel becomes hypomineralized and white spots appear on the teeth. You can't really get fluoride naturally from food, so be sure baby is getting it in his water or a vitamin supplement. And if you filter your water with a Brita or Pur, don't worry—those types of filters don't remove fluoride (although more sophisticated filters that use reverse osmosis, deionizers, or activated alumina *can* remove it).

***

Wow, we covered a lot in this chapter! But I hope that now you feel more confident and comfortable about getting started with feeding baby and providing a safe eating environment for your little one. Also, I hope that I've answered some questions that may have been weighing on your mind—about things like gluten, GMOs, and organic food.

Now we can jump into Part II, where you can get cooking! Before we dive into planning out baby's first meals, we'll cover some basics: those essential nutrients that baby needs to get in the first two years of life to ensure that he's developing to his full potential.

PART II

What to Feed Your Baby & Toddler: A Month-by-Month Guide

3

Key Nutrients Babies Need

The nutrition your baby receives will serve as the building blocks of good health for the rest of her life. The appropriate intake of nutrients is essential to cognitive and social development, physical growth, maintaining healthy body weight, resisting infections, and improving resistance to those nasty little bacteria that can make us sick.

But how do you make sure that your baby is getting the proper nutrition? What does he need to have proper balance? Aside from the obvious issue of teeth and chewing ability (which baby will gradually acquire), is it different from the types of foods that adults (or even older kids) are supposed to eat?

The purpose of this chapter is to describe the essential nutrients, as well as what they do and, most important, which baby-friendly foods contain them. You may find some of this chapter a bit nerdy and dense. I am including all of this detail, though, because if you are at all like me, you might wonder what some of these words that we see associated with health mean (like, *riboflavin* sounds healthy, but what the heck is it?!). Unless you were a nutrition major, you might not recall what many of these nutrients actually do. So think of this as a refresher in basic human nutrition—or a crash course!

Remember, it is necessary for baby to have a balanced diet, so it's critical to know which nutrients are important and which good foods you can give him to make sure he is healthy. In chapters 4 through 6, I give a more detailed month-to-month plan for incorporating foods that are rich in many of these nutrients into baby's diet and at which months of age they are especially important to consume.

Vitamins and Their Functions

VITAMIN	ALSO KNOWN AS	KEY FUNCTIONS
A	retinol activity equivalents (RAE)	Tissue and skin health, vision, cell and bone growth
B1	thiamine	Conversion of food into energy; healthy skin, hair, and heart; healthy nervous system; efficient digestion; proper muscle development
B2	riboflavin	Conversion of food into energy, nervous system health, possible reduction of inflammation, protection against cancers
B3	niacin	Healthy skin and nails, mobility, DNA metabolism and cell communication, cognitive functioning
B5	pantothenic acid	Cell function, hormone and cholesterol production
B6	pyridoxine	Macronutrient metabolization, formation of new red blood cells, neurotransmitter development
B7 (or H)	biotin	Cell growth and repair; skin, hair, and nail health; digestion
B9	folate	Blood cell and protein production; digestion
B12	cobalamin	Healthy nerves; red blood cell and DNA formation
C	ascorbic acid	Healthy immune system, tissue growth and repair, bone and tooth development, blood vessel health, prevention of cell damage
D	calcitriol	Calcium and phosphorus maintenance, healthy bones and teeth, brain and nervous system, muscle movement
E	y-tocopherol	Antioxidant, muscle growth, visual and neurological function
K	phytonadione	Blood clotting, heart health, strong bones
Choline		Nervous system health, metabolism regulation, liver health

Minerals and Their Functions

MINERAL	KEY FUNCTIONS
Calcium	Strong bones and teeth, heart and muscle health
Chloride	Cell health, blood volume and pressure, body fluid pH
Chromium	Fat and carbohydrate metabolism, brain function
Copper	Metabolism; bone, tissue, brain, and heart health
Fluoride	Tooth-decay prevention, bone-structure maintenance
Iodine	Cell metabolism, thyroid function
Iron	Red blood cell and energy production, metabolism and growth
Magnesium	Energy production, metabolism of macronutrients, bone and muscle health, digestion
Manganese	Metabolism, bone and tissue development, free radical protection
Molybdenum	Enzyme and cell function
Phosphorus	Bone and tooth development, metabolism, cell and tissue repair
Potassium	Cell health, blood pressure, electrical conduction in the body, muscle functioning, digestion, brain and nerve functioning
Selenium	Thyroid health, DNA synthesis, cell protection, bone health
Sodium	Balance of the body's fluids, nerve and muscle function
Sulfur	Cell and tissue health, enzyme function, protein synthesis
Zinc	Immune system support, production of proteins and DNA, wound healing, smell and taste support

What Happens if Baby Becomes Nutrient Deficient?

As we learned in chapter 1, you don't need to be underweight to be malnourished. Although most infants in developed countries are well fed (meaning they get enough calories), many commonly have nutrient deficiencies from poor diet choices. Iron deficiency is fairly common in toddlers and may cause anemia and delay development. Other common deficiencies are vitamin D (which we typically get from the sun, not food), fiber (a lack of which can lead to constipation), and omega-3 fatty acids. In the United States, most deficiencies aren't due to poverty or disease; they develop because parents don't know the importance of the nutrients or know what early symptoms to look for. In fact, you may not even realize your child is deficient in a nutrient because sometimes there *are* no overt signs, and pediatricians don't routinely test for deficiencies unless there is medical cause for concern. But not to worry; a healthy, balanced diet can reverse deficiencies and protect against their health effects. Given our relatively affluent and increasingly inactive lifestyles, caloric requirements are too often met with high-fat and sugar-rich foods, and we don't eat enough dietary fiber, fruits, and vegetables. This can have a number of detrimental effects on the health of toddlers and infants, including dental caries (aka cavities), constipation, and obesity.

MACRONUTRIENTS VS. MICRONUTRIENTS? ─────────

In brief, *macronutrients* are carbohydrates, fats, and proteins; *micronutrients* are vitamins and minerals. We need more macronutrients, but micronutrients are also needed in small quantities to ensure critical functioning of our bodies. Most vitamins we need are not produced by our bodies (or produced only in very small amounts), so we obtain them from food or the environment.

Which Nutrients Does Your Baby Need?

Now let's review the macro- and micronutrients that your baby needs to grow healthy and strong. I will discuss the macronutrients first, followed by the micronutrients. This is a pretty exhaustive list, and I will provide some ideas on food sources that are high in each nutrient, so you can be aware of foods that might be good to build into baby's diet. In chapters 4 through 6, I will highlight nutrients that are important at specific points in baby's development and also give you some more specific baby-friendly food options and delicious recipes you can try to ensure baby is getting all that she needs to grow healthy and happy.

Carbohydrates

Baby Needs: For babies 6 to 12 months old, aim for about 95 g/day of nutritious carbohydrates (not candy!). For babies 13 to 24 months old, try for 130 g/day.

Why Baby Needs It: Babies, like humans at every stage of life, need carbohydrates to provide fuel for their bodies. Carbohydrates are the energy that fuels baby's metabolism; they are used by your baby's nervous system, kidneys, muscles, and brain for efficient functioning. Carbohydrates are also key for the process of eliminating waste efficiently, and they help baby's body maintain the right balance of hormones (like glucagon and insulin) to properly regulate blood sugar.

There are two types of carbohydrates: simple and complex. Simple carbohydrates are called that because they have just one or two sugars. Examples of foods that contain simple sugars include fruits (which have fructose and/or glucose as sugars), some vegetables (which can contain maltose), and milk products (which can contain lactose). Table sugar (sucrose) is also a simple carbohydrate, often found in foods such as soda, candy, and syrups. These types of carbohydrates can be broken down and used easily by the bacteria in the gut. In contrast, complex carbohydrates are often considered better for the body because the sugar molecules are arranged in long, complicated chains that are less likely to be used first by bacteria, and leave more to be absorbed. Additionally, the nutritional value of many foods that contain simple carbohydrates, like soda and candy, is very low (note that this is *not* the case for all foods that contain simple sugars—fruits and veggies, for example, are highly nutritious). While carbohydrates have a place in baby's diet, eating too much of them can have a negative effect if it means that baby is not eating enough protein, fat, and other essential nutrients.

Where Baby Can Get It: Nutritious, complex carbohydrates can be found in whole grains, beans, and starchy vegetables like corn and peas, as well as potatoes (just not french fries and other deep-fried potato snacks!). Each of these foods is also likely to provide vitamins and minerals that are important for maintaining health.

Carbohydrates are highlighted as the nutrient of month 7; see page 93 for more information and additional meal ideas, including good sources of carbohydrates for baby.

Fat

Baby Needs: For babies 6 to 12 months old, aim for 30 g/day of fat (with 4.5 g coming from omega-6 fatty acids and at least 0.5 g coming from omega-3 fatty acids). However, the total daily fat grams needed after age 1 have not been determined. According to the Institute of Medicine, 30 to 40 percent of total calories should come from fat. For example, if your toddler's weight suggests he needs approximately 1,000 calories, 300 to 400 of those calories should be coming from fat. Since there are 9 calories per 1 gram of fat, this equals about 44 grams of fat per day.

Why Baby Needs It: Your baby needs healthy fats to grow and develop. Fats provide baby's body with energy and help support her growth, brain development, and healing of wounds. Fats also help your baby's organs by cushioning them and regulating temperature. Baby also needs fats in her diet to increase absorption of fat-soluble vitamins, such as vitamin A and vitamin D. It is recommended that you feed your baby fatty fish at least twice a week to ensure adequate intake of essential fats, such as omega-3 fatty acids, for brain development.

EPA AND DHA: WHAT ARE THEY?

Many studies have shown the health benefits of consuming the two main omega-3 fatty acids, EPA and DHA. Benefits includes healthy brain development, improved memory, and improved cognitive and intellectual abilities in childhood and later in life. While feeding baby a meal of fish might not seem that appetizing, it can be! Baked salmon (wild-caught, not farmed), trout, canned light tuna, and pollock are all great low-mercury options; for a full list, you can refer to the Smart Seafood Buying Guide produced by the Natural Resources Defense Council (NRDC; www.nrdc.org/stories/smart-seafood-buying-guide). Just make sure there are no small bones in the pieces! For an omega-3-rich meal for your toddler, check out the recipe for Salmon Sticks on page 169.

You may be concerned that your baby will become overweight or even obese if she eats fats, but that concern is unfounded. Fats are an important part of a healthy diet. Consuming the right amount of healthy fats, like omega-6s and omega-3s, is crucial for growth and development. In fact, the American Academy of Pediatrics recommends avoiding *any* fat restriction before the age of 2 years. This doesn't mean you should allow baby to pig out on the cookies. It is important to limit foods that are known to be sources of unhealthy saturated and trans fats (like store-bought cakes and pastries), since they can pose health risks later in life. About 40 percent of your baby's energy comes from fat, and her body will store any excess.

Where Baby Can Get It: Good sources for healthy fats include salmon, dark poultry meats, dairy products like whole milk, and produce like avocados.

Fats are highlighted as the nutrient of month 9. Check out page 101 for additional information on fat and more ways in which you can get healthy versions of it into baby's diet.

Protein

Baby Needs: For babies 6 to 12 months old, aim for 1.6 to 2.2 g/kg (grams per kilogram of weight) of protein per day. Babies 13 to 24 months old need 1.2g/kg per day. (The conversion ratio is 2.2 pounds = 1 kg.) So if your 11-month-old weighs 21 pounds (or 9.5 kg), he needs between 15 and 21 grams of protein each day. And if your 18-month-old weighs 24 pounds (or 10.9 kg), he needs 13 grams of protein each day.

Why Baby Needs It: All cells are made of protein, and protein is essential for the constant process of cell repair and rebuilding. Protein is the basic building block for muscles and other body tissues, and is necessary for the development of bones, skin, cartilage, and blood. Proteins provide energy, but to be used by the body they must be broken down into their simplest components (amino acids). Some amino acids are nonessential, which means your baby's body can make these for itself (in other words, they don't have to come from food). Other amino acids are found only in food and are essential to a healthy body. If baby does not consume these essential amino acids, her body will not be able to repair damaged tissue or maintain its cells. Unlike carbohydrates and fat, protein is not stored in the body. Since there are no protein reserves to draw upon, your baby must eat sufficient protein *each day*.

Where Baby Can Get It: Good sources for your baby include animal (red meats, poultry, fish, casein, and whey) and vegetable proteins (such as soy). However, not all proteins are created equal, and they are ranked by their biological value, a measure of how well the protein your baby consumes is integrated into his body. Protein sources with the highest biological value include milk, soybeans and soy milk, eggs, cheese, rice, quinoa, beef, and fish. Another method used to evaluate protein is the protein digestibility-corrected amino acid score (PDCAAS), which indicates how well your body can digest the protein. Foods with high rankings on the PDCAAS scale include milk, egg whites, soybeans, beef, chickpeas, black beans, fruits, vegetables, and legumes. As you can see, there is quite a bit of overlap between the two, making it easier for you to choose foods for your baby that are both high in biological value as well as readily digestible.

Protein is highlighted as the nutrient of month 15. See page 128 for more ideas on baby-friendly sources of protein.

ARE ALL PROTEINS THE SAME?

While most people have no problem getting enough protein, it is important to note that not all protein is the same. Consuming *complete* or high-quality protein can be tricky. *Complete protein* sources are foods containing all the essential amino acids in "perfect" proportions—amounts optimal for your body to support its functions. Most animal foods have complete protein (for example, eggs, milk, cheese, fish, poultry, meat), whereas plant foods (such as nuts, seeds, grains, beans) tend to lack one or more amino acids. Does that mean you should focus only on animal foods? No. Baby can get all needed protein by eating plant foods *if* he eats a variety. While they are considered incomplete because they lack one or more of the essential amino acids, combining complementary proteins (two or more protein sources that together contain all the essential amino acids, such as rice and beans) can provide baby with all the essential amino acids. Further, complementary proteins don't need to be eaten within the same meal; baby will absorb everything just fine if he eats them within the same day. Ideally, you should try for baby to get a balanced mix of both animal and plant proteins, because in addition to the protein, baby is also getting vitamins and minerals from them, and a balance between the two is key.

There are fourteen different vitamins and sixteen different minerals, each of which carries out various functions in the body and is required for overall well-being. Here, I'll cover many of these that are particularly important for baby's development.

Vitamin A

Baby Needs: The amount of vitamin A in food is measured in mcg RAE, which stands for microgram retinol activity equivalents. (These can be converted to international units or IU, but scientists seldom use this term.) Babies 6 to 12 months old need 400 to 500 mcg RAE/day. Babies 13 to 24 months old need 300 mcg RAE/day.

Why Baby Needs It: Vitamin A is needed to keep tissue and skin healthy—that is why you may often see it included in skin-care products (like retinol). It is also vital for maintaining baby's vision; deficiency can lead to night blindness—the inability to see correctly at night or in low light). Vitamin A is also needed for cell growth and has an important role in bone growth.

Where Baby Can Get It: Vitamin A is commonly found in plants that range in color from yellow to red. Good sources for babies include soft carrots, sweet potatoes, butternut squash, cooked spinach or kale, small pieces of bell peppers (even green ones!), broccoli (pureed, or tiny, well-cooked stalks for toddlers who are ready), peas, and scrambled eggs. Fruits like peaches, mangoes, and cantaloupe are also good sources of vitamin A. Many baby cereals are now fortified with vitamin A. In most developed countries, breast milk contains enough vitamin A for the first 6 months of life (unless the mother is deficient herself).

FOOD FOR THOUGHT It is important that baby get the correct amount of vitamin A. Very high amounts can be toxic, but the amount of vitamin A found in most plant foods, like peaches or carrots, is safe for baby. Getting too much vitamin A from fruits and vegetables may cause the skin to become yellowish, but it's not a sign of toxicity and will gradually fade with reduced intake. However, it can be possible to get too much vitamin A from animal sources, like liver. But don't skip foods that contain vitamin A for fear of baby getting too much. It is far more common to be deficient than to overdo it, and a deficiency in this vitamin has been linked to immunodeficiency diseases, respiratory illnesses, and diarrhea. Just have baby pass on the liver paté for now!

Vitamin A is highlighted as the nutrient of the month 8; see page 97 for more ideas on how you can incorporate it into baby's diet.

Vitamin B1

Baby Needs: A baby 6 to 12 months old needs 0.17 mg/day. A baby 13 to 24 months old needs 0.5 mg/day.

Why Baby Needs It: Vitamin B1, also known as thiamine, is essential in the process of converting food into energy, and it is also necessary for healthy skin, hair, and heart. Thiamine is also vital to keeping baby's nervous system functioning. It provides energy to baby's brain, keeps digestion efficient, and ensures that muscles develop properly. In short, thiamine is used nearly throughout the body for its most important functions.

It is difficult to consume too much thiamine, because it is a water-soluble vitamin. This means that whatever the body doesn't use will be passed through the urine. It is possible, however, to get too *little* thiamine, and this can pose serious consequences for baby's development. Thiamine deficiency can result in beriberi disease (once common; now rare in the United States), which can affect a baby's heart and circulatory system or damage a baby's nerves.

Where Baby Can Get It: Good sources of thiamine include fortified pastas or baby cereals (baby-friendly powdered versions of grains, such as oatmeal, that you can thicken with water, breast milk, or baby formula), flax seed, acorn squash, avocados, peas, yogurt, watermelon, brown rice, and some animal sources, such as chicken, pork, or oily fish. Many legumes, such as navy beans, are also good sources of thiamine. Try to avoid polished white rice; thiamine (as well as many other healthful nutrients!) is lost in the processing, which removes the germ as well as the bran.

Vitamin B1 is the nutrient of month 23, so check out page 162 for ideas on how to incorporate this vitamin into baby's diet.

Vitamin B2

Baby Needs: For babies 6 to 12 months old, aim for 0.4 mg/day. Babies 13 to 24 months old need 0.5 mg/day.

Why Baby Needs It: Vitamin B2, or riboflavin, is another B vitamin needed to convert food into usable energy. It also has a role in maintaining baby's nervous system. Additionally, scientists are studying riboflavin for its ability to protect against certain cancers and reduce inflammation in the body. Consuming the right amount of riboflavin also supports the functions of the other B vitamins. Like thiamine, riboflavin is water-soluble, making it very unlikely to cause toxicity. Getting too little riboflavin can affect baby's vision and cause dermatitis or migraines, and deficiency is more common than many people realize. Not to worry; a number of healthy foods provide riboflavin, so there is little risk that your baby will be deficient in riboflavin as she starts solid foods.

Where Baby Can Get It: Good sources of riboflavin include fortified cereals, spinach, broccoli, and animal products like chicken, salmon, dairy, and eggs. Here are a few examples of foods that are rich in vitamin B2: 1 cup cooked pureed spinach (0.43 mg; make creamed spinach by adding some milk for additional vitamin B2), 1 hard-boiled egg (0.26 mg), ½ cup steamed broccoli (0.12 mg).

Vitamin B2 isn't highlighted as a nutrient of the month, but that doesn't mean it isn't important for baby. Many foods that are rich in vitamin B2 are also rich in other highlighted nutrients, so you will likely have no problems making sure baby gets her recommended amount.

Vitamin B3/Niacin

Baby Needs: For babies 6 to 12 months old, aim for 4 mg/day. For babies 13 to 24 months old, aim for 6 mg/day.

Why Baby Needs It: Just like thiamine and riboflavin, vitamin B3 (or niacin) is important for baby's nervous and digestive systems, as well as developing healthy skin and nails. Because of the role that niacin plays in developing strong muscles and bones, it is essential for mobility. It is also involved in DNA metabolism and communication between cells. Researchers are also studying niacin for its abilities to lower low-density lipoprotein (LDL; bad) cholesterol. Niacin is important for cognitive performance, since it is involved in brain-cell functioning. For most children in developed countries, there is little risk of niacin deficiency. However, children who do not get adequate amounts of niacin can develop skin lesions or swelling, particularly in and around their mouths and tongues. Niacin deficiency is also associated with pellagra, a disease characterized by ulcers, skin inflammation, and diarrhea. Too much niacin (from over-the-counter or prescription niacin use) has been linked to muscle pain, gout, skin flushing, and digestive distress. As with the other B vitamins, it is difficult to consume too much niacin via food, as it is also water-soluble.

Where Baby Can Get It: Good sources of niacin for baby include almost all animal proteins (like chicken, fish, and pork) as well as sweet potatoes, squash, peas, beets, mushrooms, and bell peppers. Many grains are fortified with niacin, including brown rice, buckwheat, and barley.

Vitamin B3 is highlighted as the nutrient of month 16, so check out page 132 for more ideas on how you can make sure baby is getting enough.

Vitamin B6

Baby Needs: Babies from 6 to 12 months old need 0.3 mg/day. Babies 13 to 24 months old need 0.5 mg/day.

Why Baby Needs It: Vitamin B6, or pyridoxine, is another important B vitamin that helps your body metabolize macronutrients (proteins, carbohydrates, and fat). It also helps to form new red blood cells, is involved in your baby's brain and nervous-system development by making neurotransmitters, and is essential to many other responses.

Where Baby Can Get It: Baby can easily get all the vitamin B6 he needs through his diet. B6 is widely available in a variety of foods; good sources are baked potato, salmon, chicken, cooked spinach, pureed prunes, chickpeas, brown rice, banana, avocado, pork loin, and nuts. (Just make sure they are pureed and thinned, and see page 37 on food choking hazards.)

Vitamin B6 is the nutrient of month 18, so check out the recipes and other food ideas on page 139.

Vitamin B9/Folate

Baby Needs: Babies from 6 to 12 months old need 80 mcg/day. Babies 13 to 24 months old need 150 mcg/day.

Why Baby Needs It: You probably heard an awful lot about the importance of folate when you were pregnant. Folate, or vitamin B9, is another B vitamin found in food, though you may have seen the synthetic version, folic acid, in many fortified foods and supplements. During pregnancy, it is particularly important that women get enough folate because it is associated with healthy neural-tube development (the beginning parts of baby's brain and nervous system). But the importance of this nutrient doesn't end with childbirth. It is particularly important for your baby's digestion because it helps form blood cells, break down nucleic acids, and produce proteins. Like the other B vitamins, folate is water-soluble, so it is difficult to consume too much; many people actually do not consume enough, which is one reason why the synthetic folic acid is supplemented in many foods. Getting too little folate can lead to a condition called megaloblastic anemia, which often leads to weakness and fatigue. It turns out that humans absorb folic acid more efficiently than folate from foods. Regularly consuming foods that are naturally high in folate or supplemented with folic acid can supply you with adequate or near-adequate amounts of the vitamin if you know where to look for it. However, since we absorb folic acid differently from folate, fortified foods and supplements containing folic acid should not be consumed in excess (higher than the upper limit of 300 mg for toddlers 1 to 2 years old) because it can hide a vitamin B12–deficiency anemia.

WHAT IS A DFE? —————————————————————————

Folate intake is expressed in dietary folate equivalent (DFE) because food-based folate and folic acid from supplements are not absorbed the same way. One microgram of food-based folate equals 0.6 micrograms of folic acid from fortified foods or supplements (if consumed with food—but only 0.5 micrograms if consumed on an empty stomach, so be sure to take supplements with food).

Where Baby Can Get It: Good sources of folate that are baby-friendly include produce, like avocados or papaya, and animal products, like beef, poultry, and eggs. Folic acid is also found in many fortified cereals.

Folate is the nutrient of month 17, so check out page 136 for more information on good food sources.

Vitamin B12

Baby Needs: For babies 6 to 12 months old, aim for 0.5 mcg/day. When your baby is 13 to 24 months old, aim for 0.9 mcg/day.

Why Baby Needs It: Vitamin B12, also known as cobalamin, helps keep baby's nerves healthy, assists with the formation of red blood cells, and helps make DNA. It is helpful for some infants with feeding difficulties, neurologic problems, and developmental delays, so it is important that your baby consume an adequate amount each day.

If you had an adequate supply of vitamin B12 during your pregnancy and your baby was full-term, he was born with a store of it large enough to last for the first eight months of his life. Like the other B vitamins, this one is water-soluble, so it is difficult to consume too much. After around 8 months of age, it is possible for your baby to suffer from deficiency if he is not eating a balanced diet. And if you were vegetarian or vegan during your pregnancy and breastfeeding, your baby may need to consume extra B12, so discuss this with your doctor. In infants, a deficiency in vitamin B12 has been linked to failure to thrive and serious difficulties in movement.

Where Baby Can Get It: Good sources of vitamin B12 include fish, meats, poultry, and eggs (if baby gets tired of scrambled, try making hard-boiled eggs and chopping them up in sizes that she can handle), as well as fortified cereals.

Vitamin B12 is the nutrient of month 11. See page 108 for additional vitamin B12-rich food ideas for baby.

Vitamin C

Baby Needs: For babies 6 to 12 months old, aim for 50 mg/day. From ages 13 to 24 months, aim for 15 mg/day.

Why Baby Needs It: You probably know vitamin C (ascorbic acid) as key for a healthy immune system, particularly if you are feeling under the weather. But vitamin C is also important for baby's tissue growth and repair, as well as the development of bones and teeth. Vitamin C assists in making collagen, a protein found in bones, blood vessels, cartilage, skin, and tendons. This vitamin also promotes healthy blood vessels and neurotransmitters in the brain. Vitamin C is considered an antioxidant and prevents damage to baby's cells, including cells in the brain. In developed countries, severe deficiency in vitamin C is rare. However, evidence suggests that many people (including babies) have low levels of vitamin C in the body. Too little vitamin C in baby's diet can lead to gingivitis; rough, dry, scaly skin; and nosebleeds. Vitamin C is water-soluble, so it is difficult to consume too much. When more than 1 gram of vitamin C is ingested in a day, the body will absorb less than 50 percent; the rest will be excreted in the urine.

Where Baby Can Get It: Good sources of vitamin C include raw fruits and vegetables. Depending on where baby is developmentally, she may not be able to handle raw fruits or veggies. Vitamin C can be lost in the process of cooking, so fresh soft fruits like berries, kiwi, and oranges, or foods such as red bell peppers and leafy greens are best. Although vitamin C is added to certain cereals, be aware that the vitamin C content degrades over time (so check expiration dates, and don't bother to stock up on cases of cereal).

Vitamin C is the nutrient of month 10, so flip ahead to page 104 for additional ideas on how you can incorporate it into baby's diet.

Vitamin D

Baby Needs: For babies 6 to 12 months old, aim for 400 IU/day. For babies ages 13 to 24 months, aim for 600 IU/day.

Why Baby Needs It: Vitamin D is known as the "sunshine vitamin" because our bodies can make it from exposure to sunlight. It helps maintain adequate levels of calcium and phosphorus, and optimal intake of vitamin D ensures that your baby's bones and teeth develop normally. Vitamin D is used by baby's body to carry messages from the nerves to the brain, and her muscles need this vitamin to move. It is easy to get too little vitamin D, and several recent studies suggest that many adults and children don't get the recommended amounts. Deficiency can lead to rickets, a condition in which children develop soft and brittle bones.

Where Baby Can Get It: Very few foods naturally contain vitamin D. Some good sources are animal products such as fatty fish (salmon, canned tuna, canned sardines, catfish) and eggs, as well as fortified foods such as milk, orange juice, margarine, and cereal. However, when choosing the latter foods, make sure to read the label—not all of them will be fortified (for example, some margarines are not). For some baby-friendly ideas, try fortified cereals (most contain 40 IU per serving), 6 ounces fortified yogurt (80 IU), 3 ounces cooked salmon (450 IU), or 1 large egg (41 IU; note that only the yolk provides the vitamin D).

Vitamin D is not a nutrient of the month, mostly because there are not a lot of specific baby-friendly foods that naturally contain it. However, between the fortified foods that you will be feeding baby, and some of my suggestions (along with those occasional rays of sunlight and possibly a supplement), baby will be able to get what he needs.

The American Academy of Pediatrics recommends regular supplements of 400 IU of vitamin D for partially and exclusively breastfed babies starting from the first several days after birth, until your baby is weaned and drinking 32 ounces of vitamin D–fortified formula or *whole* cow's milk. The same goes for babies who are fed less than 32 ounces of vitamin D–fortified formula a day. It is also recommended for babies who live in areas that get little sunlight (such as far-northern countries and northern states in the United States where the daylight hours are short in winter, or urban areas where sunlight is blocked by buildings and air pollution). Babies with medium to dark complexions need even more exposure to sunlight than those with fair skin, but too much sun exposure leads to increased risk of sunburn and some skin cancers. Talk with your doctor to ensure that your baby receives an adequate amount of vitamin D. It can be tricky to safely get it from the sunlight in kids younger than 2 years. Baby's tender skin can't safely be in the sun unprotected for longer than a few minutes, and it is not recommended to apply sunscreens on babies younger than 6 months of age. And to make matters even more difficult, baby doesn't get the benefits of vitamin D from the sun if sunscreen is applied.

Vitamin K

Baby Needs: For babies 6 to 12 months old, aim for 2.5 mcg/day. For babies 13 to 24 months old (whose newborn injection has worn off), aim for 30 mcg/day.

Why Baby Needs It: Your baby may have received an injection of vitamin K immediately after birth. This is standard practice because babies are born with low levels of vitamin K, which is integral to helping blood clot. Without this injection, some babies develop vitamin K–deficiency bleeding. This vitamin remains important even after baby's birth, however, and especially as he starts eating solids. Vitamin K is an essential micronutrient because it helps blood clot, but it also keeps your baby's heart healthy and helps build strong bones.

Where Baby Can Get It: Good sources of vitamin K include green leafy vegetables, vegetable oils like soy and canola oils, avocado oil (which is preferred due to its added health benefits), cabbage (cooked and pureed), and broccoli (pureed, or cooked stalks for the older kids), cucumbers (pureed or in very small pieces), and prunes (pureed). Try preparing your baby's green leafy vegetables with some fat (such as oil) to improve absorption.

Vitamin K is the nutrient of month 22. So be sure to check out page 159 for additional recipes that will boost baby's vitamin K levels.

Calcium

Baby Needs: For babies 6 to 12 months old, aim for 260 mg/day. For babies 13 to 24 months old, aim for 700 mg/day.

Why Baby Needs It: Calcium is best known as the foundational nutrient for strong bones and teeth. But other organs need calcium, including your baby's heart. Calcium works with vitamin K to ensure sufficient blood clotting, and it helps your baby's muscles develop and function. It is also needed for secretion of the parathyroid hormone as well as nerve signaling. Adequate intake of calcium is also essential for your baby's long-term health, protecting against bone-weakening disorders such as osteoporosis.

Where Baby Can Get It: Good baby-friendly sources of calcium include many commonly eaten foods. You probably know that dairy products—such as milk, yogurt, and cheese—are rich in calcium, but there are many nondairy sources, too. Your baby can get adequate calcium from fortified foods, like cereals, as well as naturally occurring calcium from greens, peas and beans, and fish such as sardines. Although the bioavailability of calcium in most greens is high, spinach is one exception due to the oxalate content. Other foods that contain a high amount of phytates, like bran cereals, may also decrease the availability of calcium. A single serving of milk (8 ounces) or plain yogurt (8 ounces) provides as much calcium as two to five servings of cabbage or broccoli—but don't skip these plant foods, as they are full of other important nutrients!

Calcium is the nutrient of month 13, so check out page 121 for additional ways to ramp up baby's calcium intake.

Fiber

Baby Needs: There is no established recommended dietary fiber amount for children less than 1 year old. For babies 13 to 24 months old, aim for 19 g/day.

Why Baby Needs It: Constipation is not fun, especially when you are a baby! However, there are ways you can help prevent it. One is to make sure that baby is obtaining adequate amounts of fluids and fiber. It is important to note that there are two types of fiber—soluble and insoluble—and each has different properties. Soluble fiber is fermented in the colon and slows down the passage of food through baby's digestive system. Insoluble fiber, as the name implies, does not dissolve in water and provides bulk in baby's colon, helps speed food transit time, and helps baby stay regular. In other words, insoluble fiber is more helpful in preventing constipation.

Where Baby Can Get It: Many fruits, vegetables, and grains are excellent sources of fiber, so if you are feeding baby a well-balanced diet, getting the right amount of fiber shouldn't be a problem. Pears, pureed prunes, strawberries, apples, and mangoes, as well as most veggies (especially winter squash, broccoli, and carrots) and beans (especially soybeans, navy, and pinto), cooked oatmeal, quinoa, and whole-grain breads, cereals, and pastas are great sources of fiber for baby. About ½ cup of vegetables or one piece of fruit provides your baby with about 3 grams of fiber. When choosing whole grains, aim for sources that have 2 to 3 grams of fiber listed on the nutrition label for each serving.

Fiber is highlighted on page 124 at 14 months; flip ahead to see additional ways in which you can be sure baby gets enough fiber.

Iron

Baby Needs: For babies 6 to 12 months old, aim for 11 mg/day. For babies 13 to 24 months old, aim for 7 mg/day.

Why Baby Needs It: For your growing baby, the mineral iron helps produce red blood cells and adenosine triphosphate (ATP), the body's energy. Iron is made up of proteins that are central to metabolism and moving oxygen from the lungs to the rest of your baby's tissues. Iron is also involved in hormone synthesis and is needed for growth. The World Health Organization estimates that the number-one nutritional deficiency across the globe is iron deficiency. Those who are severely iron deficient may become anemic. Fortunately, you gave your baby a 6 months' supply of iron during pregnancy. After reaching that age, your baby will need sources of iron in his diet.

You may have noticed that many cereals are fortified with some micronutrients, such as iron. This is done by the food companies because, after 6 months, babies have depleted the iron stores they built up while developing in the womb and need to start getting iron from food. That can be challenging for those starting solids. This puts babies at risk for iron deficiency, which has been associated with developmental delays. And it turns out that breastfed babies are most at risk. Breast milk contains iron, but just not enough of it. So commercially available cereals are fortified with iron to help make sure babies are getting enough. However, baby can get iron from other sources, such as meat, poultry, fish, and seafood, which all contain iron that is easily absorbed.

Where Baby Can Get It: There are two good sources of iron in food—heme and non-heme. Heme iron comes only from animal foods, such as meats, poultry, and seafood (clams contain nearly 14 mg in a 3-ounce serving!). It is the better absorbed form of iron, with a 15 to 35 percent absorption rate. Non-heme iron exists in both animal and plant foods and is found in fortified cereals, eggs, milk, lentils and other legumes, spinach, and prunes. However, most of the iron in these foods is poorly absorbed. Many foods that contain non-heme iron, like beans and grains, also contain phytates, which bind to iron and prevent the absorption. Not to worry, though! There are several ways you can bump up your baby's ability to absorb non-heme iron. Serve these foods alongside others that are rich in vitamin C, such as lentils with red bell peppers, or a fresh-fruit dessert after a legume meal. Strawberries, papayas, kiwi, oranges, cantaloupe, and guava are all packed with vitamin C! You can also increase the absorption of non-heme iron from plants by serving it alongside meat or fish, and try cooking with a cast-iron skillet—the iron from the cookware will leach into the food.

Iron is our first nutrient of the month, for month 6, so be sure to check out the ideas starting on page 88 for boosting baby's iron levels.

Magnesium

Baby Needs: For babies 6 to 12 months old, aim for 75 mg/day. For babies 13 to 24 months old, aim for 80 mg/day.

Why Baby Needs It: More than 300 enzymes require magnesium for normal functioning. Magnesium is necessary for energy production and is implicated in the metabolism of fats, proteins, and calcium. Although magnesium is not the first mineral that comes to mind when thinking of bone health, it plays a crucial role in maintaining your baby's bone structure. Magnesium aids in tissue repair, nerve impulses, and muscle function, as well as moving stool through the intestine. It also aids in the regulation of blood sugar and blood pressure. Magnesium deficiency is associated with increased inflammation and oxidative stress, diabetes, kidney disease, and osteoporosis. Fortunately, your baby can get all the magnesium he needs from a variety of foods.

Where Baby Can Get It: There are many excellent baby-friendly food sources that are high in magnesium, including legumes, like black beans, and vegetables such as broccoli and spinach. Nuts and seeds are also great sources, especially almonds, cashews, and peanuts; try making nut butters that are thin enough for baby to handle or swirl them into another dish. But remember, never feed a baby or toddler whole nuts or seeds because she can too easily choke on them. Since food processing removes a lot of the magnesium naturally present in the germ and bran of grains, processed foods are often fortified with magnesium, including many breakfast cereals. Tap and mineral water also contain magnesium. A good rule of thumb is that foods high in fiber are also typically high in magnesium.

Magnesium is our last nutrient of the month, for month 24, so flip ahead to page 167 for more food ideas on boosting baby's magnesium levels.

Manganese

Baby Needs: For babies 6 to 12 months old, aim for 600 mcg/day. For babies 13 to 24 months old, aim for 1.2 mg/day.

Why Baby Needs It: Manganese is a mineral needed for baby's brain to function normally. It plays a role in metabolism, is needed for bone and connective tissue formation, and even helps with detoxification by fighting free radicals. Manganese is sometimes added to supplements with other minerals like calcium and vitamin D to prevent osteoporosis. Deficiency can lead to poor growth and disruption of fat and carbo-hydrate metabolism. While certain minerals like calcium and phosphate, as well as phytates, can decrease the body's ability to absorb manganese, the good news is that deficiency is rare and there are plenty of healthy sources that provide adequate amounts for your baby.

Where Baby Can Get It: Manganese is found in most grains and nuts. Meat, fish, and chicken are also good sources. Certain beans, such as lima beans, navy beans, and pinto beans, also contain manganese. Breast milk contains manganese, with a higher bioavailability compared to formula. Although spinach and sweet potatoes are good sources of this mineral, oxalic acid present in these foods may decrease absorption (although cooking the foods can help because it breaks down oxalic acid).

Manganese is the nutrient of month 20, so be sure to check out the recipes and information beginning on page 152.

Potassium

Baby Needs: For babies 6 to 12 months, aim for 700 mg/day. For babies 13 to 24 months, aim for 3 g/day.

Why Baby Needs It: Your baby's body uses potassium to maintain proper electrolyte and fluid balance in the cells, which helps keep blood pressure healthy. Potassium is used to conduct electricity in the body and helps muscles contract. This mineral also aids in digestive functions like breaking down carbohydrates and is necessary for controlling the body's pH balance. In addition, potassium is involved in major brain and nerve functions.

Potassium is found in many foods, but if a baby's diet doesn't include enough of them, she can become deficient. When there are very low levels of potassium in the blood, a condition called hypokalemia can cause issues with your baby's heart and kidneys. Preterm infants who are born small for gestational age are at increased risk of hypokalemia. On the other hand, it is possible for babies to get too much potassium, leading to hyperkalemia—excessive blood levels of potassium. This condition is most common in babies who were born with an extremely low birth weight. For the most part, healthy babies with healthy diets get adequate potassium from their foods.

Where Baby Can Get It: Good sources of potassium for babies include sweet potatoes, cooked winter squash, cooked lentils, bananas (pureed, or cut into appropriate-size pieces), and cow's milk. In general, fresh fruits, dairy, meats, and vegetables are all rich sources of potassium, and processed foods usually have less potassium than fresh, whole foods.

Potassium is the nutrient of month 19, so flip ahead to page 148 to read about additional ways in which you can increase baby's potassium levels with the right foods.

Selenium

Baby Needs: For babies 6 to 24 months old, aim for 20 mcg/day.

Why Baby Needs It: Selenium is necessary for your baby's thyroid to function normally, and it plays an important role in DNA synthesis. Selenium also protects cells from oxidative damage and is needed for optimum bone health as well as blood-sugar control. Although deficiency is very rare, low levels are associated with diabetes and cancer. Scientists have been investigating whether additional selenium supplementation is beneficial for cognitive and thyroid function as well as better glucose control.

Where Baby Can Get It: Seafood, particularly halibut and sardines, is one of the best sources of selenium. Other good sources include cereals, dairy (such as cottage cheese), eggs, and Brazil nuts (just make sure to chop them up small enough or puree to a "butter"). Although many plant-based foods contain selenium, the actual content varies depending on the soil in which the plants were grown.

Selenium is the nutrient of month 21. Check out page 155 for additional ways to include selenium-rich foods in baby's diet.

Zinc

Baby Needs: For babies 6 to 24 months, aim for 3 mg/day.

Why Baby Needs It: Zinc is an essential mineral that your baby needs for his rapidly dividing cells, for protein and DNA synthesis, and for numerous other changes taking place in his tiny body as he develops. It's involved in more than a hundred different enzymatic systems! Zinc is also essential for motor function. Without enough zinc, your baby may become anemic, his wounds may heal slowly, he may be at increased risk for failure to grow at a normal rate and an altered sense of taste, and he could develop diarrhea or even pneumonia. Zinc is needed to fight infection, so it's important to make sure your baby is getting enough, especially when transitioning from breast milk to solid foods. Zinc deficiency is common throughout the world; some estimates suggest that about 17 percent of the global population may be at risk. Fortunately, your baby can get all the zinc needed fairly easily from a well-balanced diet.

Where Baby Can Get It: Good sources of zinc include fortified breakfast cereals; ground lamb, beef, and turkey; Alaskan king crab (be sure to cut it small); tofu (after 8 months of age, baby's digestion can handle it; when cut into small cubes, it is a great soft finger food to try); chickpeas and kidney beans; wheat germ and whole grains; yogurt and milk; and collard greens, just to name a few!

Zinc is the nutrient of month 12, so be sure to check out some additional zinc-infused recipes you can make for your baby-turning-toddler beginning on page 111.

FOOD FOR THOUGHT The human body absorbs less zinc from nonanimal sources than from animal sources. However, you can increase the amount of zinc absorbed by soaking and cooking legumes (or buying the canned variety) and combining plant-based zinc sources with acidic ingredients such as lemon juice.

SUMMARY OF BABY'S KEY NUTRITIONAL NEEDS FROM AGES 6 TO 24 MONTHS

Following is a quick and handy list of the important nutrients that your growing baby needs as you start introducing solids. Included are some easy sources for these nutrients.

Summary of Baby's Nutritional Needs from
Ages 6 to 24 Months

NUTRIENT	AMOUNT NEEDED PER DAY	SOME FOOD SOURCES
Vitamin A	6 to 12 months: 400 to 500 mcg RAE 13 to 24 months: 300 mcg RAE	Bell peppers, breast milk, broccoli, butternut squash, cantaloupe, carrots, cereal, eggs, kale, mangoes, peaches, peas, spinach, sweet potatoes
Vitamin B1	6 to 12 months: 0.17 mg 13 to 24 months: 0.5 mg	Acorn squash, avocados, brown rice, chicken, flax seed, fortified cereals (including oatmeal) and pastas, legumes (like navy beans), oily fish, peas, pork, watermelon, yogurt
Vitamin B2	6 to 12 months: 0.4 mg 13 to 24 months: 0.5 mg	Broccoli, chicken, eggs, fortified cereals, salmon, spinach
Vitamin B3	6 to 12 months: 4 mg 13 to 24 months: 6 mg	Barley, beets, bell peppers, brown rice, buckwheat, chicken, fish, mushrooms, peas, pork, squash, sweet potatoes
Vitamin B6	6 to 12 months: 0.3 mg 13 to 24 months: 0.5 mg	Avocado, banana, brown rice, chicken, chickpeas, pork loin, potato (baked or boiled), prunes, salmon, spinach
Vitamin B9	6 to 12 months: 80 mcg 13 to 24 months: 150 mcg	Avocado, beef, eggs, fortified cereals, papaya, poultry
Vitamin B12	6 to 12 months: 0.5 mcg 13 to 24 months: 0.9 mcg	Eggs, fish, fortified cereals, meats, poultry
Vitamin C	6 to 12 months: 50 mg 13 to 24 months: 15 mg	Kiwi, leafy greens, oranges, red bell peppers, some cereals, strawberries
Vitamin D	6 to 12 months: 400 IU 13 to 24 months: 600 IU	Eggs; fatty fish; fortified cereals, milk, and yogurt; some margarine
Vitamin K	6 to 12 months: 2.5 mcg 13 to 24 months: 30 mcg	Broccoli, cabbage, cucumbers, green leafy vegetables, oils (such as soy, canola, avocado), prunes
Calcium	6 to 12 months: 260 mg 13 to 24 months: 700 mg	Beans, cheese, cow's milk, fortified cereals, greens (but not spinach), peas, sardines, yogurt

Fiber	13 to 24 months: 19 g	Apples; mangoes; most vegetables and legumes; oatmeal (cooked); pears; prunes; quinoa; strawberries; and whole-grain breads, cereals, and pastas
Iron	6 to 12 months: 11 mg 13 to 24 months: 7 mg	Fish and seafood (clams), fresh fruits after legumes, lentils with red bell peppers, meats, vegetables alongside a meat or fish
Magnesium	6 to 12 months: 75 mg 13 to 24 months: 80 mg	Breakfast cereals, broccoli, high-fiber foods, legumes (such as black beans), nut butters (such as almond, cashew, peanut), spinach, tap and mineral water
Manganese	6 to 12 months: 600 mcg 13 to 24 months: 1.2 mg	Beans (such as lima, navy, pinto), chicken, fish, meat, most grains and nuts, spinach, sweet potato
Potassium	6 to 12 months: 700 mg 13 to 24 months: 3 g	Bananas and other fruits, dairy, lentils, meats, vegetables
Selenium	6 to 24 months: 20 mcg	Brazil nuts (smoothed to make a butter), cereals, cottage cheese, eggs, halibut, sardines
Zinc	6 to 24 months: 3 mg	Alaskan king crab; chickpeas and kidney beans; collard greens; cow's milk; fortified cereals; ground beef, lamb, turkey; tofu; wheat germ; whole grains; yogurt

***

Whew! That is a *lot* of information, but I bet you know more than you ever thought you would about nutrition for your baby. We have covered the key nutrients for a healthy baby, *why* they are key, and *where* you can find them, and now we can begin to delve into chapters 4 through 6 (which is where the fun really begins, because you start actually feeding baby). These three chapters are designed to take you and baby through ages 6 months to 2 years, month by month, so that you can see how your baby is developing both physically and cognitively, and also learn ways you can support her growth through good nutrition!

This certainly doesn't mean that your baby needs to eat *all* of the foods discussed here or in the next section *every* day. Remember that most foods baby consumes contain multiple nutrients. For example, cooked lentils contain folate, iron, fiber, manganese, protein, and vitamins B1 and B6, in addition to nutrients we didn't even talk about, like copper and pantothenic acid, helping baby get part of his daily dose of all of these nutrients. The goal here is to try to offer foods that are healthful and wholesome and contain diverse nutrients that we know will be beneficial to your baby.

CAN'T I JUST GIVE BABY VITAMINS AND NOT WORRY ABOUT ALL OF THIS?

The American Academy of Pediatrics does not typically recommend a multivitamin supplement for healthy babies and toddlers who eat a variety of foods and are growing normally. However, some pediatricians suggest that you put your baby on a liquid vitamin supplement, since doing so does not seem to pose any increased risk. This is not a bad idea, especially if you are nursing and your diet isn't perfect (whose is?), plus baby will need that vitamin D boost. Also, if you live in a place where the water isn't fluoridated, then you will likely need to put baby on a supplement to get her the fluoride she needs to prevent cavities; beginning at 6 months, when baby teeth start emerging. Being on a vitamin supplement doesn't mean that baby doesn't still need to eat a balanced diet, though. Remember, half of the goal is to develop a sophisticated palate and enjoy diverse, nutritious foods. This will help with food choices and preferences later in life. So if you can combine healthy eating with a multivitamin supplement, you will be covering all of your bases, and the days that baby doesn't eat so well will balance out with the days you accidentally forget to give her that supplement! If you choose to give your baby a vitamin supplement, make sure that it does not provide megadoses or an excess of any nutrient, and if it's one that is designed to makes kids want to take it—like gummies—keep them out of baby's reach.

If you are looking for a supplement, I recommend Rainbow Light. They launched a new pre- to post-natal-targeted multivitamin line to support the first 1,000 days of mom and baby, beginning with pre-conception nutrition. In it, they've included a formula for infants and toddlers—NutriStart Plus—made with organic fruits and vegetables (which is also non-GMO and gluten-free).

4

Starting Solids (6 to 12 Months)

Congratulations! You have made it through the first 6 months of parenting. It isn't always easy, but as I am sure you are starting to see, it gets easier, especially as your baby becomes more active and interactive with you. One of the most memorable times you will have is baby's first meal. So get the camera out, and let's go! (Just remember, keep it low-key. You want baby relaxed and open to the new experience, not overwhelmed by paparazzi.)

This chapter will cover feeding baby solids from ages 6 months to 1 year. Since during this time baby is eating mostly purees, and parents and caregivers are feeding her, you can have a lot of fun with trying out different tastes and combinations. This chapter introduces what is happening with baby developmentally during this time. I touch on the basic milestones, but note that the "normal" age ranges for these are very broad. Baby development and milestone achievement is *a lot* more variable than fetal development (which is pretty similar for most healthy *in utero* babies from week to week), so this overview is just meant to give you an idea about what is happening or will happen soon. Don't stress if you baby isn't doing some of these things yet. He likely will any day or week now. Every baby develops at a slightly different pace. Some are early crawlers or walkers, and others hit these milestones a little later. But if you are worried at all about baby's progress, be sure to bring it up with your pediatrician.

The primary focus of this section is to introduce each month's nutrient of the month. It is important that baby have a well-rounded diet to get all of the nutrients she needs. And what better way to learn about how to do that than to highlight one each month so you can learn about which foods are best to incorporate into baby's diet to make sure she doesn't become deficient in anything? This chapter also lists foods high in each nutrient that you can include in baby's diet, along with some specific amounts to give you some context. In addition, for each month, I'll offer a few fun and easy-to-prepare recipes.

> **FOOD FOR THOUGHT** The USDA has a great website that contains nutrition information for all of the food products out there. So if you are wondering how much iron is in the serving of peaches you are about to feed your little one, you can look it up! Check it out: https://ndb.nal.usda.gov/ndb/

We have already covered some of the practical details, such as how much food baby needs and how thick the food should be at first, back in chapter 2. So if it's been a while since you read it, flip back for a refresher before you actually start feeding baby. There, I outline how much baby needs to eat at different stages, and I offer a lot of practical tips on getting started with feeding your baby solid foods.

> **FOOD FOR THOUGHT** Remember, you should avoid foods your baby could choke on, including popcorn, raw vegetables and hard fruits, whole grapes, raisins, and nuts. Don't forget, baby has no teeth yet (or only a few). He needs to learn to chew (masticate) the food with his gums and teeth and then be able to easily swallow it; so the softer, the better. You need to avoid giving food in a size that could block baby's airway. Check out page 36 for more important information on preventing and responding to choking.

What Is Happening Developmentally? An Overview

Before getting into the nitty-gritty of feeding your baby, let's take a moment to consider what is going on developmentally from 6 to 12 months. Not only is your baby growing rapidly in size, but her mind is quickly evolving, and she is acquiring new skills almost daily.

> **FOOD FOR THOUGHT** Considering that your baby is just starting to get a grasp on things—no pun intended—eating food on his own might still be a difficult task. It is important to find a balance between feeding your baby with a spoon and allowing him to experiment with grabbing food and bringing things to his mouth. One trick that worked for me (twice!) is to let baby have a spoon to hold, while you

feed him with another spoon. Remember, early on, baby just wants to mimic what he sees you doing, so having a spoon to hold will make him happy! Later, as he gains more control over his motions, you can experiment with letting baby feed himself (just be prepared for the mess!).

WHAT IS BABY-LED WEANING?

Perhaps you've heard of a concept known as "baby-led weaning," or BLW. With BLW, the idea is that your baby does all the work so you can forgo purees and weaning spoons and simply let your baby feed himself with finger foods. In theory, this sounds great—it means you can be more relaxed about feeding, and maybe even enjoy a meal yourself at the same time as your baby, since she is eating little bits of whatever you are eating. However, I do *not* think this is a wise practice to follow for babies between 6 and 12 months. Your little one is still in the process of learning how to use all of her new skills (like bringing food to and from her mouth and sitting up on her own). Plus, think about what you eat. Tiny bits of "adult" food that aren't the proper consistency for baby can be hard to handle digestively, and they can pose a greater risk of choking. Also, unless you are a super-healthy eater yourself, letting baby eat what you're eating might mean she gets more processed foods than she should. BLW has been associated with insufficient calorie intake, high salt intake, and inadequate iron intake—all of which can be detrimental to your baby in the long run. I do think there is a place for this practice later on, but it needs to be done safely and when baby is ready. If you are keen on BLW because of the idea of bringing the family together, note that many of the recipes that follow are family friendly. Think about it, if you add a dollop of crème fraîche to the Zucchini-Pea Puree with Mint recipe on page 92, I bet your significant other will think it is some fancy soup recipe you're trying out.

From 6 to 12 months, as your baby develops mentally, emotionally, and physically, she is constantly gaining new skills that allow her to explore the world in different ways (such as shaking, banging, poking, and dropping things). She is becoming much stronger and more independent.

By the time she reaches 12 months, your baby's relationship with food has expanded beyond just being able to feed herself from a variety of healthy options provided by you. Now her relationship with food is strongly influenced by external factors like the eating environment and the presence of others at mealtimes. Not only is a 12-month-old likely able to drink from a cup and take things out of containers and put them back in, but she can also respond to simple requests and copy behavior that she sees. She tries to say words you say and mimics your gestures at the table. The key point here: a *lot* will be happening during these 6 months. Not only will you be training baby to eat healthy, nutritious foods, but you will also be establishing her food etiquette and manners. If you haven't already, now is the best time for you and the rest of the family to begin modeling good eating behavior for your child.

WHICH FOODS SHOULD YOU START WITH? ——————

This is really up to you. Most parents opt to start with a cereal, but there's no rule that says you have to. You can start with vegetables if you like. However, as you will soon see, there is good reason *not* to skip the cereal.

Getting Started

Chapter 2 covered a lot of the details about getting started with feeding baby, so here I list just a few key points that are worth noting again.

- Between the ages of 6 and 12 months, baby is still getting all of his necessary nutrition and calories from breast milk and/or formula. You introduce foods during this time not for nutrition but more for fun and trying to get baby to like the taste of healthy foods. This is why foods during this phase are referred to as *complementary*. Solid foods complement the nutrition that baby is getting from breast milk or baby formula.

- In chapter 1, I noted that it can take up to 8 days to get a baby to prefer a taste, so don't give up too easily or move on to the next food too quickly. For example, if you start with peas, try feeding your baby only peas (as the complement to breast milk or formula) for a week. He may or may not like something on the first try, but slow and persistent exposure is key to teaching him to accept solids and the actual food itself.

- Be mindful of the texture and thickness. Remember, baby is used to liquid, so whatever you feed him should be close to a liquid consistency when you start. You can gradually offer thicker textures and at some point add small, soft chunks, but for now the texture should be very thin (you can thin out fruits and veggies with formula, breast milk, or water).

- Don't ever force anything on your baby, whether it's a particular food she doesn't like or the food she's lost interest in before finishing all 4 ounces that you've prepared. Keep in mind that it is essential to respect your baby's internal hunger cues. You can always take a break and try again later if baby seems fussy or disinterested in eating.

- Don't forget that growing infants learn by copying, and research shows babies are more likely to eat foods they see their parents eating. So try to eat with baby to model behaviors you want to see from him.

What's in Store?

Within a few months of introducing complementary solids, you should be able to feed your baby a variety of foods, in addition to breast milk or formula, such as meats and fish, fruits, vegetables, cereals, and eggs. As your baby develops, you will also be able to start moving on from purees to finger foods that are cut into small pieces, soft, and easy to swallow. You'll want to wait until your baby is capable of sitting upright on her own and successfully bringing objects (like food) to her mouth, usually around 9 months or so. By 12 months, you should not be spoon-feeding your baby any more at all. It's essential to time your introduction of finger foods according to your baby's development and mastery of basic self-feeding skills. Introducing your baby to finger foods before she is ready may increase the risk of choking and not taking in adequate amounts of food (see baby-led weaning on page 83). Some good early finger foods to try are cut-up banana; scrambled eggs; chopped-up hard-boiled eggs; well-cooked whole grains; pasta; well-cooked and chopped-up (ground) meats like chicken, lamb, or beef; and well-cooked veggies that are soft and easy to chew, like squashes, potatoes, and mushy carrots. You can also mash foods with a fork or blend them in a blender.

Last but not least, I want to emphasize again that it's never too early to teach your child good eating habits. This includes, first and foremost, exposing your baby to a wide variety of fruits, vegetables, whole grains, lean meats, eggs, and dairy. In addition, baby needs to learn the actual process of eating. I don't mean just learning how to use a spoon or a cup, but also coming to recognize her own hunger cues, practicing good manners, and eating in a healthy mealtime environment.

HOW TO CREATE A HAPPY (AND HEALTHY) MEALTIME ENVIRONMENT

There is so much more to raising a healthy child than just food! Here are a few ideas.

- Have your baby eat meals with you and the whole family whenever possible.

- Make mealtimes a pleasant, sharing experience.

- Eat a wide variety of wholesome foods yourself; baby takes cues from you.

- Limit TV/screen/digital media time during mealtimes, and encourage baby to pay attention to eating and enjoying her food.

- If you have older kids, make it a rule: We sit when we eat (no running around playing and coming to the table just to graze). That way, baby doesn't feel like she's missing out on fun because she is strapped into a chair. Also, running around while eating is a leading cause of choking on food.

- As your baby begins to understand you more, practice good manners and set appropriate boundaries for mealtimes.

DOES ORDER MATTER?

Considering the connection between early feeding and food preferences later in life (flip back to page 12 for more on this), you may be wondering, "If I feed my baby sweet foods like fruits, will he develop a dislike for vegetables right away?" The answer is no! The order in which you introduce foods will not affect your child's preferences. With early feeding, it's not necessarily about the order; it's about the variety and types of food you choose to give your little one, and the repetition. The health benefit of feeding baby a naturally sweet fruit is much different from (and far better than) feeding baby salty, mashed up french fries with sugary ketchup. And remember, as discussed previously, if baby seems to dislike the taste of a veggie or new food, you can pair it with a sweet fruit that she likes, and eventually be able to condition her to not need the fruit.

WHAT ABOUT FOOD ALLERGIES?

If you are nervous about feeding baby because you are concerned about food allergies, you aren't alone. Food allergies are a scary concern for most, if not all, parents. It certainly makes the introduction of new foods a stressful time, not knowing if your baby could have a potentially life-threatening response. Flip ahead to page 183, which covers this topic in detail and offers advice on when you need to be alert to whether baby has allergies, and the stages when you should introduce foods that are common allergens (like peanuts or cow's milk), based on the latest scientific findings.

What to Feed Your Baby: A Month-by-Month Guide for 6 to 12 Months

Now that we've tackled some of the basics on beginning to feed your baby (again, refer back to chapter 2 for details on how much to feed baby, how often, and so on), let's travel through the first 6 months of feeding your little one, month by month, to see how you can help baby grow big and strong by focusing on foods that are rich in the nutrients needed during this period. Throughout the rest of this chapter, I will highlight nutrients of the month and suggest a few foods rich in certain nutrients that are critical at this point to introduce to baby's diet. I provide some recipes for each month, as well as suggestions for ways to ensure baby gets plenty of the needed nutrients.

There are several reasons why I list so many foods for each month, even though I advise giving baby each new food for 8 days before moving on to another one. First, this is a guide, and you are the master chef for your baby. I offer several options each month so you can pick and choose what you think baby would like (you know her best). Second, not all foods will require 8 days of exposure to get baby to accept them. She's likely to embrace sweeter fruits more quickly than many vegetables and more tart fruits (so baby may love ripe pears, but balk at apricots at first). If you find that baby really seems to like a food, there's no need to wait more than 3 days before trying something new. You do, however, want to wait *at least* 3 days to determine whether baby has a reaction to the food (say, an allergic reaction on her skin or a bad diaper rash). If, for example, you try several new foods at the same time, and baby develops a bad diaper rash, you won't know which food may be the culprit.

At the end of each chapter in this part, I include sample menus for baby that incorporate some staple foods, as well as some of the delicious recipes included here. This way you will have lots of ideas for healthy ways to make sure baby is getting exposed to all of the nutritious foods he needs.

WHAT'S HAPPENING?

Pumping Iron. By 6 months, your baby already has a wide skill set in terms of social and emotional development, language and communication, cognitive skills, and motor skills. These include behaviors such as responding to other people's emotions, looking at himself in the mirror, starting to bring things to his mouth, and showing curiosity about items that are out of reach. He can typically respond to a voice by turning toward it, and he's even started to make repetitive vowel-consonant combinations ("goo-goo, ga-ga" is practice for "da-da" or "ma-ma"). Many babies will be upset if you take away a toy that they like, and they will work to get a toy they want by reaching for it. In terms of motor/physical development, your 6-month-old is just starting to be able to sit without support (just keep the pillows nearby, as he still tends to topple over sometimes), and he is gaining more control over his hands, like being able to pass items back and forth and put them in his mouth (which is why you need to keep small toys and other items out of reach). He may even be able to bear some weight on his legs. At this point, your baby is developing skills that go hand in hand with timing the introduction of complementary foods. As I've mentioned, what better time to start introducing new foods than when your baby is eager (and able) to explore?

NUTRIENT OF THE MONTH: IRON

Iron is necessary for red blood cell production and the transport of oxygen throughout the body. As mentioned on page 72, babies are born with some iron stored in their bodies, and just as it is for adults, maintaining those iron stores is important for feeling and functioning at their best. Although breast milk has some iron, it is not enough to keep up with the demands of rapidly growing infants, and infants who are breastfed exclusively are at risk of iron deficiency if complementary feeding is not introduced at 6 months. Babies with a deficiency may experience slow weight gain, slower development, and irritability, accompanied by pale skin and a poor appetite.

For adults and older kids, it is relatively easy to get adequate iron from food. Iron is abundant in animal foods (red meat, poultry, seafood) and plant foods (dark leafy green vegetables, beans, dried fruits), as well as iron-fortified breads and pastas. However, since baby is new to eating solids and not exactly ready to order a hamburger, your best bet for this month is to focus on her getting iron from fortified cereals.

In addition to commercially available baby cereals (which are iron forti-fied), you can also make sure baby gets plenty of iron by offering him foods like peas or peaches, as well as trying the recipes that follow. Beans (cooked well, then pureed and thinned with breast milk, formula, or water) are also a great source of iron, but notice if they make baby gassy and uncomfortable. Tip: If you are using canned beans, rinse them thoroughly with water before serving; this flushes away a lot of the carbohydrates that we can't break down that can cause gas. Some additional ideas to get more iron in baby include 1 cup pureed white beans (8 mg), ½ cup pureed lentils (3 mg), and 3 ounces ground lamb, pureed (2.3 mg). Other great sources of iron are mentioned on page 73.

BABY OATMEAL

MAKES ABOUT ½ CUP

Oats are a great grain to start with because they are naturally high in iron. You can process rolled oats (not quick-cooking or instant) into a fine powder in the blender or food processor for a smooth fiber- and mineral-rich baby cereal that you can mix with fruit or vegetable puree as baby is introduced to more foods.

¼ cup rolled oats
⅔ cup water

Put the oats in a blender or food processor and process to a fine powder.

Bring the water to a boil in a small saucepan over medium-high heat. Whisk in the oatmeal powder and lower the heat. Cook, stirring continually, until the water is absorbed and the cereal is thickened and smooth, 1 to 2 minutes. (If it's too thick, thin with a little cool water, breast milk, or formula.) Let it cool to room temperature before feeding baby.

Make ahead: Process a few cups of oats at a time and store the powder in a jar so that you can quickly cook individual portions. For toddlers and older kids, you can process the powder a little more coarsely and use this instead of quick-cooking oats, which have been processed to remove their nutritious outer hull, or instant oats, which often have lots of added sugar.

BABY BARLEY CEREAL

MAKES ABOUT ¾ CUP

Barley is an iron-rich, nutty-tasting grain packed with fiber and a variety of other important nutrients. It is a nice change from rice cereal or oats, and it pairs deliciously with savory foods like veggies or Zucchini-Pea Puree with Mint (page 92). Use a powerful blender to grind the dry barley into a fine powder.

¼ cup pearled barley
1 cup water

Put the dry barley in a blender or food processor and process to a fine powder, 3 to 4 minutes.

Bring the water to a boil in a small saucepan over medium-high heat. Whisk in the barley powder and lower the heat. Cook, stirring continually, until the mixture is smooth, about 5 minutes. (If it's too thick, thin with a little cool water, breast milk, or formula.) Let it cool to room temperature before feeding baby.

Make ahead: You can grind up a few cups of the barley powder in small batches and store it in a jar in the refrigerator so that you can cook single servings of cereal quickly. When you want to prepare a serving, use 1 part barley powder to 3 parts water.

ZUCCHINI-PEA PUREE WITH MINT

MAKES ABOUT 1½ CUPS

Make baby's first blend a nutritional powerhouse! Lightened up with summer squash (zucchini), sweet green peas make an iron-, folate-, and vitamins C and K–rich puree for baby. A brief steaming preserves the vegetables' nutrients and bright color.

1 medium zucchini, washed and ends trimmed
1 fresh mint leaf
1 cup fresh or frozen sweet green peas

Slice the zucchini into 1-inch rounds. Tear the stem and center rib from the mint leaf.

Bring an inch or so of water to a boil in a pan fitted with a steamer. Place the zucchini in the steamer, cover, and steam until tender, 6 to 7 minutes. Transfer to a food processor.

Place the peas in the steamer, cover, and steam until tender, 5 to 6 minutes for fresh and about 2 minutes for frozen. Spoon the peas into the bowl of the food processor. Let the vegetables cool to room temperature.

Add the mint leaf to the vegetables and process to a smooth puree, adding a few tablespoons of water as necessary to get a smooth consistency before feeding baby.

To store: Refrigerate for up to 2 days or freeze individual portions for up to 3 months.

BLENDS?

You may be wondering when it is okay to start mixing foods. The answer is: right away! While most people start off feeding baby single-food purees, that isn't really necessary. I advise starting with a few single-food purees; then you can branch out with blends and others mixtures. Remember, blending different fruits and vegetables can enhance the taste and make it easier for baby to develop a liking for some of those more bitter (yet oh-so-nutritious) vegetables.

WHAT'S HAPPENING?

Peekaboo! The games have officially begun! By this age, your baby actively engages in hiding games, and you may find yourself playing peekaboo pretty regularly throughout the day. Baby finds it absolutely fascinating that you can cover an object and he can "find" it. Baby is also more sensitive to the nuances of tones, so if you raise your voice, don't be surprised if baby cries.

Physically, baby can most likely sit unassisted at this point (if he can't, don't worry—he'll get there at his own pace). And many babies are on the move, via either creeping, crawling, or rolling around on their bellies all over the house.

NUTRIENT OF THE MONTH: CARBOHYDRATES

Make sure baby gets enough of the healthy carbohydrates she needs to keep up with her increasing activity. Carbohydrates are the primary fuel for infants, and you don't want baby running on empty! As noted on page 59, carbohydrates are needed not only to maintain proper hormonal balance but also to assist in proper energy balance. The proper balance of carbohydrates helps your baby sustain her energy level evenly throughout the day, so she isn't going from sugar rush to sugar crash. And with all the energy baby is using now, we want to make sure to keep up a steady supply!

It is easy to make sure baby gets enough carbohydrates; the challenge is to make sure these are from healthy, nutritious sources. Try to opt for fruits and vegetables in addition to cereals as carbohydrate sources. That way, baby is getting plenty of other nutrients, and also trying out new tastes.

Some baby-friendly higher-carbohydrate foods include 1 cup cooked, pureed oatmeal, unsweetened (30 g); 1 cup cooked, pureed brown rice (45 g); ½ cup mashed and pureed sweet potatoes (15 g); ½ cup well-mashed (or pureed) chickpeas (15 g); 1 medium (the size of a baseball) pear or apple, pureed (15 g); ½ pureed ripe banana (15 g); 1 cup whole-grain baby cereal (15 to 20 g); and ½ cup steamed and pureed peas (10 to 15 g).

In addition to getting carbohydrates from these healthy sources, try the following recipes.

SMOOTH SWEET POTATO PUREE

MAKES ABOUT 1 CUP

Sweet potatoes are packed with healthy carbohydrates, as well as vitamins A, B6, and C. Their naturally sweet flavor and creamy texture make them an appealing early choice for baby. Once baby gets used to the flavor of sweet potatoes on their own, mix sweet potato puree with a little apple or pear puree.

Bake several sweet potatoes at once so that you (and the rest of the family) can enjoy them for lunch or dinner, too. (For adults and older kids, try them sliced lengthwise and topped with black beans, salsa, a spoonful of yogurt, and a squeeze of lime.)

One 8- to 12-ounce sweet potato

Preheat the oven to 400°F.

Scrub the sweet potato well with a vegetable brush under running water. Prick in several places with a sharp paring knife, then place on a baking sheet or pan. Bake until very soft when you pierce it with a knife, 45 to 60 minutes. Let cool to room temperature.

Slice the sweet potato in half lengthwise, scoop the cooked potato from the skin, and place in the bowl of a food processor. Process until smooth; add a little water as necessary to get a smooth consistency. (Discard the skin or, since it is so nutritious, you may want to use as shells to stuff for an older kid or an adult.)

When baby is ready to handle a little more texture, you can mash the sweet potato coarsely with a fork, and eventually graduate to offering her small soft pieces to feed herself.

To store: Refrigerate for up to 3 days or freeze individual portions for up to 3 months.

APPLE-PEAR PUREE

MAKES ABOUT 2½ CUPS

Apple-pear sauce is full of healthy carbohydrates and vitamin C, and it's sweet and easy on the tummy. Mix it with a little rice cereal, baby oatmeal, or barley cereal for variety.

1½ pounds pears
1½ pounds apples

Peel and core the pears and apples and cut them into 1-inch chunks.

Bring an inch or so of water to a boil in a pan fitted with a steamer. Place the chunks in the steamer, cover and steam until the fruit is very soft when you pierce it with a knife, 6 to 8 minutes. Let cool.

Transfer the fruit to a blender or food processor and puree until smooth, adding a few tablespoons of water as necessary to get the right texture.

To store: Refrigerate for up to 3 days or freeze individual portions for up to 3 months.

BANANA MASH

MAKES ABOUT ½ CUP

Naturally sweet and creamy, and conveniently portable, bananas are an ideal choice for one of baby's first foods. They're packed with potassium and carbohydrates and C and B vitamins. Choose ripe bananas; they're sweeter and softer to mash. As baby grows, you can make this puree chunkier; eventually you can give baby small cubes of banana. Banana mash doesn't store well, so make small batches for baby to eat that day.

1 ripe banana

Peel the banana and break into chunks. Place in a bowl and mash well with a fork. Add water if needed to thin the mixture to the right consistency before feeding baby.

CARROT-CHICKPEA MASH WITH CUMIN

MAKES ABOUT 1 CUP

Chickpeas are a super-legume: they're packed with healthy carbohydrates, folate, protein, and iron. Blending chickpeas with carrot is a nice way to introduce baby to their mellow, nutty flavor. When baby is old enough for dipping pita triangles, this mixture will make a great dip brightened up with a spoonful of olive oil, a squeeze of lemon juice, and a pinch of salt.

2 small carrots, peeled and cut into ¼-inch rounds
½ cup drained canned or cooked dried chickpeas
⅛ teaspoon cumin

Bring several inches of water to a boil in a pan fitted with a steamer. Place the carrots in the steamer, cover, and steam until they are very soft when you pierce them with a knife, about 10 minutes. Let cool.

Combine the carrots, chickpeas, and cumin in a blender or food processor and pulse to a smooth puree. Add a few tablespoons of water as needed to get the right consistency before feeding baby.

To store: Refrigerate for up to 3 days or freeze individual portions for up to 3 months.

WHAT'S HAPPENING?

Now You See Me; Now You Don't! Remember those days when you could put baby on the floor and know he would stay put? Those days are pretty much gone now. Baby is on the move, and that means he is getting his hands on more and more things around your house (and thus is encountering more germs).

Speaking of "seeing," baby is now seeing the world a lot more clearly. When he was born, he saw the world in shades of gray, but now his vision has developed and his eyes are working together to judge distance and focus on tasks. You may even notice that baby's irises are changing color at this point. (For some, those baby blues weren't meant to last.)

NUTRIENT OF THE MONTH: VITAMIN A

Keeping baby healthy is every parent's top priority. Page 63 outlined why having baby consume a diet that is adequate in vitamin A not only is important for growth but also helps combat infections. Vitamin A is a powerful anti-oxidant, important for cell growth and differentiation, vision, and immunity. Foods rich in vitamin A include fish oil, orange vegetables (sweet potato, pumpkin, squash, carrots), spinach, apricots, and fortified cereals. Some additional options for getting baby enough vitamin A include ½ baked sweet potato (about 700 mcg RAE), ½ cup well-cooked carrots (about 460 mcg), 1 large hard-boiled egg (75 mcg), 1 cup cooked and pureed black-eyed peas (66 mcg), and 3 ounces salmon (60 mcg).

In addition to trying the vitamin A–rich foods noted here and previously, your baby can get it from these delicious dishes.

CANTALOUPE-NECTARINE PUREE

MAKES ABOUT 1½ CUPS

Summer brings an abundance of fresh fruits with plenty of vitamins A and C, like nectarines and sweet cantaloupe. Make this tangy fruit puree in the peak of the season when fresh nectarines and cantaloupe are sweet and juicy. Substitute peaches or plums for nectarines, if you have them. Sweet honeydew melon and tart kiwi fruit are another good combination; the kiwi can be peeled and pureed without steaming.

1 ripe nectarine, halved and pitted
1 cup cubed cantaloupe

Bring about an inch of water to a boil in a pan fitted with a steamer. Place the nectarine in the steamer, cover, and steam until the fruit is soft when you pierce it with a knife and the skins are loose, 5 to 7 minutes. Let cool. Remove the skin with a sharp paring knife.

Place the nectarine and cantaloupe in a blender or food processor. Process until smooth before feeding baby.

To store: Refrigerate for up to 3 days or freeze individual portions for up to 3 months.

MANGO-BANANA PUREE

MAKES ABOUT ¾ CUP

Sweet juicy mango is likely to be one of baby's early favorite fruits. This smooth, tropical blend offers baby vitamin A, along with potassium, fiber, and vitamins C and B6. Look for mangoes that are heavy for their size and fragrant and yield to gentle pressure. Banana puree doesn't store well, so make small batches for baby to eat that day.

½ ripe mango
½ ripe banana

Peel, pit, and cube the mango. Peel and slice the banana. Place in a blender or food processor. Process until smooth, adding a little water as needed to get the right consistency before feeding baby.

what to feed your baby & toddler

BUTTERNUT SQUASH PUREE

MAKES ABOUT 3 CUPS

Orange-fleshed winter squashes, including butternut, are naturally sweet and full of vitamin A and important antioxidants. But don't stop at butternut! Other good choices are the green-skinned Japanese pumpkin, kabocha, and its reddish-orange cousin, kuri squash. All have dense, sweet flesh that makes a smooth, versatile puree. Avoid your typical American jack-o'-lantern pumpkin, as most varieties are watery and stringy. Also, canned pumpkin puree is very highly processed, and it is much tastier to prepare your own with a delicious winter squash.

1 winter squash (about 1½ pounds)

Preheat the oven to 375°F.

Using a large sharp knife, cut the squash in half lengthwise. Scoop out the seeds and place the halves cut-side down in a baking pan. Add about ½ inch of water to the pan and cover with aluminum foil.

Bake until the squash is very soft when you pierce it with a knife, 45 minutes to 1 hour. Let cool completely. Scoop out the flesh from the rind and transfer to a blender or food processor. Process until smooth before feeding baby.

To store: Refrigerate for up to 3 days or freeze individual portions for up to 3 months.

MASHED KABOCHA SQUASH
WITH PEAR AND CINNAMON

MAKES ABOUT 3 CUPS

Pear and winter squash make a hearty pairing that's packed with vitamins A and C and fiber.

1 small kabocha squash
1½ pounds pears
⅛ teaspoon ground cinnamon

Preheat the oven to 375°F.

Using a large sharp knife, cut the squash in half lengthwise. Scoop out the seeds and place the halves cut-side down in a baking pan. Add about a ½ inch of water to the pan and cover tightly with aluminum foil.

Bake until the squash is very soft when you pierce it with a knife, 45 minutes to 1 hour. Let cool completely.

Meanwhile, peel and core the pears and cut them into 1-inch chunks.

Bring several inches of water to a boil in a pan fitted with a steamer. Place the pears in the steamer, cover, and steam until the fruit is very soft when you pierce it with a knife, 6 to 8 minutes. Let cool completely.

Scoop out the squash flesh from the rind. Place the squash and pears in a blender or food processor with the cinnamon. Process until smooth, adding a few tablespoons of water as necessary to get the right consistency before feeding baby.

To store: Refrigerate for up to 3 days or freeze individual portions for up to 3 months.

---

9 MONTHS

WHAT'S HAPPENING?

Growth Spurt. By 9 months, you may notice your baby is showing a wider variety of emotions, such as fear around strangers and affection toward familiar adults. Your baby likely has favorite toys and even understands the meaning of "No." She's also finding it easier to handle food—it's likely that your little tot can seamlessly pass things back and forth between her hands and more successfully pick up little pieces of food with her thumb and index finger.

NUTRIENT OF THE MONTH: FAT

Passing objects between both hands isn't as easy as it looks. You need brains to do it. And the fuel for your brain comes from fats. You have probably heard a lot about your child needing omega-3 fatty acids DHA and EPA for proper brain development and function. It is so true! Here are two baby-friendly sources of these healthy fats you might want to try: ½ avocado (15 g heart-healthy fat), or 1 tablespoon creamy (not crunchy) peanut butter swirled into a baked apple or other pureed fruit (8 g, with 25 percent of the total fat being polyunsaturated). Note: It is best to mix nut butter with other soft foods at this age, as the texture may still be too thick for baby to handle. For more information on why baby needs fat in her diet, as well as other sources, refer back to page 60.

You can also get fats from the healthful sources in these recipes.

PEACHES AND CREAM YOGURT

MAKES ABOUT 1 CUP

As baby branches out into new flavors, give ripe peaches a try, mixed with healthy fat–rich whole-milk yogurt for added calcium, protein, and vitamin B12. Mixing your own yogurt and fruit is a good way to offer baby a chance to get used to the flavor of fruit yogurt without all the added sugar of commercial types. This recipe makes more than enough for you and baby to share, or store for a second meal.

1 ripe peach, halved and peeled
½ cup plain whole-milk yogurt
A few drops alcohol-free vanilla extract (optional)

Bring an inch or so of water to a boil in a pan fitted with a steamer. Place the peach in the steamer, cover, and steam until the fruit is soft when you pierce it with a knife and the skins are loose, 4 to 6 minutes. Let cool.

Use a sharp paring knife to remove the peach skins. Mash the peach with a fork to the consistency that's right for your baby. Spoon the yogurt into a bowl and stir in the vanilla (if using). Top with the peach.

To store: Refrigerate for up to 2 days or freeze individual portions of mashed peach for up to 3 months.

WHEN CAN YOU START YOGURT?

You may have heard from your pediatrician that baby should not have cow's milk until after age 1 year. But what about yogurt? Between 7 and 8 months is a good time to introduce yogurt to baby. Even though it is made from cow's milk, yogurt is gentler on baby's tummy due to the probiotics it contains, which make it more digestible. Opt for the full-fat variety (remember, babies need fat for brain development), as this is considered "good" fat, and avoid ones with added sugars. Yogurt naturally contains sugar (lactose), but many fruit-added yogurts also have added sugar that your baby does not need. If your baby does not like the plain variety, try adding your own pureed fruit to a plain full-fat yogurt. Also, you can experiment with different textures, like Greek or Icelandic yogurt, which are strained and so much thicker (and higher in protein!); just make sure it isn't too thick for your baby to handle.

AVOCADO MASH

MAKES ABOUT ⅓ CUP

Avocados are a nutritional powerhouse, high in healthy monounsaturated fats, vitamin E, and folate. Avocado mash won't store well, so make yourself a snack and spread any remaining on toast and top with a slice of tomato, a drizzle of olive oil, and a pinch of sea salt, then enjoy.

½ medium ripe avocado, halved and pitted

Scoop the flesh of the avocado from the peel into a bowl and mash well with a fork. Add water (or formula) if needed to thin the mixture to the right consistency before feeding baby.

BROCCOLI-POTATO CHOWDER
WITH WHITE CHEDDAR CHEESE

MAKES ABOUT 4 CUPS

This quick hearty soup starring vitamin K–rich broccoli is a source of vitamin C and folate. Baby will benefit from the healthy fat in the cheese.

1 tablespoon olive oil
½ cup finely chopped yellow onion
Pinch of sea salt
4 cups low-sodium chicken broth, vegetable broth, or water
¾ pound Yukon gold or other yellow potatoes, peeled and diced
¾ pound broccoli florets, roughly chopped
¼ cup grated sharp white cheddar cheese

In a medium saucepan over medium heat, warm the olive oil. Add the onion and salt. Lower the heat and stir frequently until the onion is soft and golden brown, 6 to 8 minutes.

Add the chicken broth and potatoes to the pan and bring to a boil. Lower the heat to maintain a simmer, cover, and cook for 5 minutes. Add the broccoli and cook uncovered for 10 minutes more, until the broccoli and potato are tender. Let cool slightly.

Transfer the soup to a blender or food processor. Process in batches until smooth; return the soup to the pot. Reheat until bubbling, then remove from the heat. Stir in the cheese until melted, and then serve.

WHAT'S HAPPENING?

Those Pearly Whites. By 10 months, baby is most likely crawling, cruising around the furniture or pulling himself up on things. It is a very active time, for both you and him! His hand-eye coordination is getting better by the day, but he still explores a lot of his world by mouth, which is why it is even more important to keep coins and other small items out of reach. And while we are speaking of mouths, baby is actively growing new teeth at this point, so we want to make sure these arrive—and remain—healthy.

NUTRIENT OF THE MONTH: VITAMIN C

Everyone knows about the immune-protecting benefits of vitamin C, so getting the right amount of it is essential to making sure baby stays healthy and fights off those nasty cold and flu viruses. Now that baby is crawling all over the place, germs are a part of life. But did you know that vitamin C is also important to growing strong teeth? Adequate levels of vitamin C keep gums healthy. However, vitamin C can sometimes be tricky to get for little ones. Oranges are known for their high levels of vitamin C, but they tend to be acidic and not very baby-friendly texture-wise. Also, if you are sticking to a no-juice regimen (which is recommended; see page 31), then you may have to get creative to make sure baby is getting enough vitamin C. Some vitamin C–packed food ideas you can try with your baby include 1 cup finely chopped ripe cantaloupe (57 mg vitamin C), ½ cup finely cut strawberries (50 mg), and ½ cup chopped ripe tomatoes (17 mg—just make sure the skin pieces are cut well). For more ideas on vitamin C sources for baby, as well as its other benefits, flip back to chapter 3.

APPLE-BEET SAUCE WITH GINGER

MAKES ABOUT 1½ CUPS

Beets may have a bad rap with some adults, but cooked baby beets are earthy and sweet. Plus they're a good source of folate, which continues to be important for brain development. Mixing beets with apple into a vibrant pink puree is a good way to introduce baby to their flavor. Also, the combination of beets and apples gives baby a healthy dose of vitamin C.

4 baby beets
2 apples
¼ teaspoon fresh grated ginger

Preheat the oven to 400°F. Remove the green tops and trim the stem ends from the beets. Scrub the beets well.

Place the beets in a small baking pan and fill the pan with about ½ inch of water, then cover tightly with aluminum foil. Bake until the beets are very soft when you pierce them with a knife, 40 to 50 minutes. Let cool and then use a paring knife to peel the beets. Cut them into halves or quarters.

Meanwhile, peel, core, and slice the apples. Bring an inch or so of water to a boil in a pan fitted with a steamer. Place the apples in the steamer, cover, and steam until soft, about 5 minutes.

Combine the beets, apples, and ginger in a food processor. Puree until smooth, adding water a tablespoon at a time as necessary for the right consistency, before feeding baby.

To store: Refrigerate for up to 3 days or freeze individual portions for up to 3 months.

ZOODLES WITH CREAMY PESTO

MAKES ABOUT 4 CUPS

Zoodles, or zucchini noodles, are a fun alternative to pasta. Gently mixed with a simple basil pesto, they make a tasty vitamin C–filled lunch or side dish that adults and older kids will like, too. A spiralizer is an inexpensive gadget that makes corkscrew-curly vegetable noodles. You can also make zucchini noodles using a vegetable peeler.

2 cups packed fresh basil leaves
¼ cup olive oil, plus 2 teaspoons
3 tablespoons water
2 tablespoons freshly squeezed lemon juice
1 small garlic clove, peeled
Sea salt
3 pounds zucchini
¼ cup grated Parmesan cheese

In a food processor, whirl together the basil, ¼ cup olive oil, water, lemon juice, garlic, and a pinch of salt until a smooth pesto sauce forms.

Rinse and dry the zucchini and trim both ends. Using a spiralizer, cut the zucchini into noodles. (If you don't have a spiral cutter, you can use a peeler to shave each zucchini into wide, thin ribbons.) Chop the pile of zucchini noodles a few times so that you have shorter strands.

In a large nonstick frying pan over medium-high heat, warm the remaining 2 teaspoons oil. Add the zucchini noodles and sprinkle them lightly with salt. Cook, stirring often, until the noodles are bright green and softened, 5 to 6 minutes.

Toss the noodles gently with the pesto sauce. Mound in bowls and cut into small pieces or mash to a texture your baby can handle. Top with the Parmesan cheese before serving.

COCONUT MILK RICE PUDDING
WITH CRUSHED RASPBERRIES

MAKES ABOUT 2 CUPS

This creamy sweet treat is made with coconut milk and topped with raspberries, which add vitamin C.

1 cup water
⅓ cup jasmine rice
1½ cups light coconut milk
2½ tablespoons sugar
1 egg yolk
2 teaspoons cornstarch
⅛ teaspoon vanilla
¼ cup fresh or thawed frozen raspberries

Place the water and rice in a small saucepan over medium-high heat and bring to a boil. Turn the heat to low, cover, and simmer until the liquid is absorbed and the rice is soft, about 20 minutes. Stir in the coconut milk and 2 tablespoons of the sugar and bring to a simmer.

In a small bowl, stir together the egg yolk, cornstarch, vanilla, and remaining ½ tablespoon sugar into a smooth paste. Whisk a little bit of the hot milk mixture into the egg mixture until smooth and then stir the egg mixture into the hot milk.

Bring to a gentle boil over medium heat. Cook, stirring constantly, allowing the mixture to bubble for 2 minutes.

Remove from the heat and spoon the mixture into bowls or ramekins. Place a piece of wax paper directly on the surface of each serving to prevent a skin from forming. Chill until cool, about 2 hours. Mash the raspberries with a fork and spoon them over the top before serving.

To store: Refrigerate for up to 2 days.

WHAT'S HAPPENING?

Warm Up the Walking Shoes. Baby is most likely getting ready to walk. Even before they walk, some babies might start to climb, so watch out if you have one of these daredevils. And babies this age love to open and close cabinets, so make sure you have these secured. Cognitively, baby is likely now showing you her budding personality, be it shy and reserved or wild and adventurous. She probably expresses her preferences for certain toys and activities. Some babies at this age look like they are entering the terrible twos, and they will cry and protest if you take them away from a toy or something they are enjoying. Some babies can even say "No" (usually not verbally yet, but by head-shaking), so you may hear (or see) that a lot. Baby is also like a sponge when it comes to language. She can understand a lot more than she can express. So be sure to continue to point out and name objects with her, as it will help her learn to speak soon. Babies at this age love to copy you, and they learn by mimicking. Whether it is brushing her hair or wiping up a spill, baby wants to do what you do, and will show you by being your little copycat!

NUTRIENT OF THE MONTH: VITAMIN B12

Babies who don't get enough vitamin B12 risk developing a deficiency. In milder cases, this can involve numbness or tingling in the hands and feet (which could affect walking); in extreme cases, this can result in severe neurological problems. Signs of deficiency tend to show up between 6 and 12 months and usually not before 4 months. Babies are at risk of a vitamin B12 deficiency if they eat little amounts of animal foods, and/or their mother was vegan during pregnancy and while breastfeeding. Vitamin B12 is abundant in animal foods, like meat, fish, and dairy, but is low in human milk and basically nonexistent in plant foods (with the exception of soy foods); this is why vegan mothers should be alert to a possible deficiency in this vitamin, and talk to their doctor about using a supplement. Here are some foods that will help get baby the vitamin B12 she needs: 3 ounces canned tuna (2.5 mcg), 3 ounces haddock (1.8 mcg), and 1 large egg (0.6 mcg) scrambled with 1 ounce Swiss cheese (1.5 mcg). If your baby doesn't like fish yet or is tired of eggs, try fortified cereals; most have 1.5 mcg per serving.

EDAMAME-AVOCADO PUREE

MAKES ABOUT 1 CUP

This mildly flavored, vitamin B12 power puree introduces baby to the flavor of edamame, which will be a favorite finger food later. Steam the edamame until very tender to get a smooth puree.

1 cup frozen, shelled, unsalted edamame
½ ripe avocado

Bring an inch or so of water to a boil in a pan fitted with a steamer. Place the edamame in the steamer, cover, and steam until the beans are soft when you pierce them with a knife and the skins are loose, 8 to 10 minutes.

Transfer the edamame to a food processor. Process, adding a few tablespoons of water at a time as needed to get a smooth consistency. Add the avocado and process until smooth before feeding baby.

To store: Refrigerate for up to 2 days.

TURKEY-APPLE PUREE

MAKES ABOUT 1 CUP

Ground turkey leg and thigh meat is a good source of protein and important B vitamins, including B12. Pureeing it with apples or sweet winter squash is a good way to introduce baby to its flavor and texture.

½ pound ground turkey
3 tablespoons water
⅓ cup applesauce

In a nonstick frying pan over medium-high heat, cook the turkey with the water, crumbling the meat with a spatula as it cooks, until it is no longer pink, 3 to 5 minutes. Let cool completely, reserving the cooking liquid.

Transfer the turkey in a blender or food processor. Process, adding as much of the cooking liquid as you need to make a smooth puree. Spoon into a bowl and stir in the applesauce before feeding baby.

To store: Refrigerate for up to 3 days or freeze individual portions for up to 2 months.

CHUNKY CHICKEN AND WHITE BEANS

MAKES ABOUT 1½ CUPS

This is an easy protein- and B vitamin–packed lunch or dinner to make when you have a cooked chicken and canned beans on hand. For babies who aren't yet ready for a chunky mixture, you can puree this mixture in the food processor until smooth.

1 boned, skinned chicken breast half (5 to 6 ounces)
1 teaspoon olive oil
1 cup drained canned or cooked dried white (cannellini) beans
½ cup chicken broth or water
1 fresh basil leaf, finely chopped

Preheat the oven to 375°F. Lightly oil a small baking pan or line it with aluminum foil.

Place the chicken in the prepared pan and drizzle with the olive oil. Bake until the chicken is opaque in the center (cut to test), about 25 minutes. Let cool completely. Use a sharp knife to slice thinly across the grain and then finely mince the slices.

Combine the beans and chicken broth in a small saucepan. Bring to a simmer and cook for 5 to 8 minutes, stirring occasionally. Mash the beans well with a fork and stir in the chicken and basil before feeding baby.

To store: Refrigerate for up to 2 days.

what to feed your baby & toddler

WHAT'S HAPPENING?

Happy Birthday! It's the *best* birthday celebration ever! You made it through the first year! Congrats! Baby is well on her way to walking and talking, and each day more and more of her personality shines through. Most 1-year-olds can stand alone, and some may have even taken those precious first few steps.

> **FOOD FOR THOUGHT** It is amazing to reflect on how much baby has grown in just one short year. His body weight has likely tripled, and his brain is approximately 60 percent of its adult size!

NUTRIENT OF THE MONTH: ZINC

Zinc is the perfect nutrient to highlight for month 12, to top off the first year of life and take your baby successfully into the second. For the first twelve months, breast milk, formula, or both should provide enough zinc to meet your baby's needs. After the first year, when it is likely that you are no longer relying on breast milk and/or formula, zinc should come from other foods, like meats, beans, dairy, whole grains, and fortified breakfast cereals. As noted on page 76, zinc is a trace mineral that plays an important role in the synthesis of DNA and RNA, and infants who are zinc-deficient can exhibit slowed growth, in addition to lethargy and delayed motor skills. Make sure baby is getting enough calories from a variety of foods to maintain a good balance of zinc. Here are some examples of ways baby can easily get the amount of zinc she needs: ½ cup wheat germ (10 mg; try mixing it with yogurt), 3 ounces ground beef (7 mg), 3 ounces shredded dark chicken meat (2.4 mg), 1 cup pureed cooked Swiss chard (0.7 mg), or 1 tablespoon tahini (0.6 mg; try this mixed with quinoa or rice).

CURRIED CAULIFLOWER-POTATO MASH

MAKES ABOUT 1 CUP

Don't overlook cauliflower! This humble vegetable may be pale but it's a surprising source of vitamins C and K, and it gives this smooth potato puree extra nutrients and flavor. Be sure to steam the cauliflower and potatoes until very tender so they are easily mashed. This delicious dish also gives baby a healthy dose of zinc from the potato.

¾ pound cauliflower florets, cut into ½-inch chunks
¼ pound Yukon gold or other thin-skinned potatoes, peeled and cut into ½-inch chunks
¼ teaspoon mild curry powder

Bring several inches of water to a boil in a pan fitted with a steamer. Place the cauliflower and potatoes in the steamer, cover, and steam until both vegetables are tender when you pierce them with a knife, 7 to 9 minutes.

Transfer the vegetables to a bowl and add the curry powder; mash until smooth—or transfer to a food processor and pulse, adding water, a few tablespoons at a time, as necessary to get the consistency you want— before feeding baby.

To store: Refrigerate for up to 3 days or freeze individual portions for up to 3 months.

what to feed your baby & toddler

BUTTERNUT SQUASH–WHOLE WHEAT SHELLS AND CHEESE

MAKES ABOUT 8 CUPS

Creamy, cheesy squash pasta? Yes, please! Winter squash adds some vitamins and sweetness to a classic macaroni and cheese recipe that is quick to make and appealing for all ages. And don't underestimate the power of the cheese, which gives baby a good amount of zinc. Mash baby's portion of these soft, saucy pasta shells to the consistency he can handle before serving.

1 pound dried whole-wheat pasta shells
1½ tablespoons butter
2 tablespoons all-purpose flour
1½ cups milk
1 cup shredded sharp cheddar cheese
⅓ cup winter squash or pumpkin puree
½ teaspoon salt
⅛ teaspoon nutmeg

Bring a large pot of lightly salted water to a boil. Add the pasta and cook until tender, 8 to 10 minutes. Drain and return to the pot.

Meanwhile, melt the butter in a medium saucepan over medium heat. Stir in the flour and cook for another minute. Slowly whisk in the milk and bring the mixture to a simmer. Cook, whisking frequently, until the sauce thickens, about 3 minutes. Remove from the heat.

Add the cheese, squash, salt, and nutmeg to the pan and stir until the cheese is melted and the sauce is smooth. Add to the pasta and mix well before serving.

HAPPY BIRTHDAY CARROT CUPCAKES

MAKES 12 CUPCAKES

Happy birthday! These cupcakes have no chunks, just moist, vanilla-flavored spice cake and tender shredded carrots. If you want to serve these as a snack, the cream cheese frosting is optional, but cream cheese is a good way to get extra zinc into baby's diet. Cooled, unfrosted cupcakes can be stored in an airtight container at room temperature for up to one day, or frozen for up to one month. Frosted cupcakes can be stored at cool room temperature for up to one day.

1½ cups all-purpose flour
1 teaspoon baking powder
½ teaspoon baking soda
½ teaspoon salt
½ teaspoon ground cinnamon
½ pound carrots, peeled and grated
2 eggs
¼ cup buttermilk
⅔ cup packed light brown sugar
¾ cup vegetable oil
1 tablespoon vanilla extract
1 recipe Cream Cheese Frosting (facing page; optional)

Preheat oven to 325°F. Line a 12-cup muffin tin with paper liners.

In a small bowl, stir together the flour, baking powder, baking soda, salt, and cinnamon.

In a large bowl, combine the carrots, eggs, buttermilk, brown sugar, vegetable oil, and vanilla. Whisk until well blended. Stir in the flour mixture until well combined.

Spoon the batter evenly into the lined cups. Bake until a wood skewer inserted into the center comes out with moist crumbs attached, 25 to 28 minutes.

Let cool in the pan for 5 minutes. Then gently transfer the cupcakes from the pan to a wire rack and let cool completely. Frost with cream cheese frosting, if desired, before serving.

CREAM CHEESE FROSTING

For a smooth frosting, be sure your cream cheese and butter are soft.

8 ounces cream cheese, at room temperature
¾ cup powdered sugar
½ teaspoon vanilla extract
2 tablespoons butter, at room temperature

In a bowl with a handheld mixer on high speed, beat together the cream cheese, powdered sugar, and vanilla until smooth. Beat in the butter until thoroughly blended. Use immediately.

***

By now, your baby is well on her way to becoming an independent eater. By following the nutritional information in this chapter, you have started her off on the right foot with her eating habits. On the following page is a trio of sample menus to help baby develop a taste for wholesome, nutritious foods. And in the next chapter, we will discuss which foods you can encourage baby to eat now that she is a toddler and ready for finger foods.

Sample Menus for Ages 6 to 12 Months

These sample menus can give you some ideas for how to combine foods for baby. Feel free to mix and match to baby's preference, as this is just a guide. Breast milk or formula *plus . . .*

ONE-DAY SAMPLE MENU—6 TO 8 MONTHS

Breakfast	Baby Oatmeal (page 90)
Lunch	Butternut Squash Puree (page 99) Zucchini-Pea Puree with Mint (page 92) 1 tablespoon Baby Oatmeal (page 90)
Snack	Apple-Pear Puree (page 95) Baby Oatmeal (page 90)
Dinner	Baby Oatmeal (page 90) Carrot-Chickpea Mash with Cumin (page 96)

ONE-DAY SAMPLE MENU—8 TO 12 MONTHS

Breakfast	Mango-Banana Puree (page 98) ⅓ cup iron-fortified cereal
Lunch	2 tablespoons well-cooked black beans ½ cup well-cooked squash
Snack	Peaches and Cream Yogurt (page 102)
Dinner	2 tablespoons boneless fish or tofu ¼ cup steamed, pureed spinach Apple-Beet Sauce with Ginger (page 105)

ONE-DAY SAMPLE MENU—8 TO 12 MONTHS

Breakfast	Mashed Kabocha Squash with Pear and Cinnamon (page 100) ⅓ cup iron-fortified cereal
Lunch	Turkey-Apple Puree (page 109) Curried Cauliflower-Potato Mash (page 112)
Snack	Coconut Milk Rice Pudding with Crushed Raspberries (page 107)
Dinner	Broccoli-Potato Chowder with White Cheddar Cheese (page 103) ¼ cup steamed peas

5

Finger Foods (13 to 18 Months)

You now have a toddler! Isn't it amazing how quickly a year can go by, and how much can happen?

This chapter will cover the basics on feeding your toddler from ages 13 to 18 months. Bye-bye purees, and bye-bye letting Mommy or Daddy control the spoon. This is a whole new ball game, and I will help you to get through it and make sure that baby (I know, he is a toddler now, but he will always be your baby) gets all the nutrition he needs. This chapter will briefly cover what is happening with your toddler developmentally during this time and then focus on a nutrient of the month that is key to baby's health. As in the previous chapter, it will also list different foods high in that nutrient that you can use to help make sure your toddler is getting what he needs to develop and thrive. In addition, a few delicious and nutritious recipes are listed for each month. And now that baby is graduating from purees to finger foods, these are recipes older kids or the whole family can enjoy.

Remember, chapters 2 and 3 covered a lot of the details on how much baby needs (calorie- and nutrition-wise), as well as offered advice and tips on making feeding baby fun! So if you need to, be sure to flip back through those chapters before trying the foods in this one.

What Is Happening Developmentally? An Overview

If you thought baby changed a lot from birth until now, wait until you see the changes that occur over the next 6 months! Physically, between ages 13 and 18 months, baby will start to walk, then run, then climb! Toddlers are active creatures, so be sure you have those baby gates secured and a safe play area for your young one to hang out. Your little one's hand-eye coordination will improve dramatically during this time, and he will be able to play with toys, puzzles, and dolls, and even be able to understand the rules for simple games (like Ring Around the Rosie, or Duck, Duck, Goose). Your toddler can understand most simple directions, making this a great time to start practicing those listening skills (like sitting in a certain spot, or waiting for Mommy to get a toy that is out of reach). Other things to look forward to include more teeth, for better chewing, and fewer naps (okay, maybe *that* isn't something you are looking forward to).

Emotionally, baby will start to express more complex feelings. Lucky for you, it will be clearer what these emotions are tied to. Baby might become emotional in response to separation from you or the loss of a toy, or she might start to show more clear signs of fear, such as crying when you want to wash her hair or when she encounters a stranger. While babies this age are still extremely egocentric, they can begin to understand simple things like the basic concepts of sharing.

Cognitively, your toddler remains a sponge and loves to mimic what he sees. Now that he is more mobile, and braver, this means he may want to do things he isn't physically ready to do independently (such as walk down the stairs or play with big sister's 5,000-piece beaded bracelet-making kit). It is important to be patient with baby and understand his frustration—and the occasional outburst over not getting his way. Just remember, these short fits are age appropriate, and a good sign that your baby is developing his emotional skill set!

Language development will also continue, and slowly, then quickly, your baby will add new words to her vocabulary. There is a lot to look forward to in these next 6 months!

Getting Started

By this point, when it comes to feeding, after working out a few inevitable kinks, you and baby are probably feeling pretty confident working together. When your little one has graduated to finger foods, you may be tempted to give him bits and pieces of your own cooked meals. This seems like a good idea because it can save you precious time that you can use for another activity outside of the kitchen. To do this, though, you may need to adjust some of your cooking methods accordingly. For example, the foods you set aside for baby should have very little added salt, and most will need to be very well cooked for baby-friendly munching and swallowing. Instead of cooking pasta in salt water, add a little salt to your dish after you serve your baby if you so desire. Be cautious about cooking with premade ingredients (like tomato sauce), which might have chemical preservatives and other additives that you wouldn't necessarily want your baby consuming. Read labels very carefully.

STORE-BOUGHT OR HOMEMADE BABY FOOD?

Not a fan of cooking? No problem! Several companies now offer a variety of delicious and healthful baby foods, so parents have a lot of options. Many are available online through delivery services or in grocery stores. Also, commercially available baby foods now come in squeeze pouches that are great for self-feeders and for babies on the go. Baby can squeeze these into his mouth (just be sure to recycle or discard the cap, as it can be a choking hazard).

The recipes included in this chapter will add more diverse flavors to baby's diet while focusing on whole, nutrient-dense foods. Because baby now can feed herself, the recipes are more geared toward allowing her to do just that. And now that baby has more teeth, she can handle a little more texture than she could in the past. I have also included suggested serving sizes for the recipes in this chapter (and the next), but remember that there is a wide variation in how much your baby eats, so this is just a guide.

EXTRA CALORIES

How many calories does baby need at this point? To briefly recap, the Institute of Medicine guidelines suggest that toddlers need between 35 and 40 calories per 1 pound of body weight per day. So if your little one weighs 20 pounds, that means he needs between 700 and 800 calories per day. Does this mean you cut baby off from eating if he is still hungry? No way! Baby should set the pace according to how much *he* needs and wants. At this age, children don't always eat the three square meals a day that we are training them for. Many times, babies will pig out at one meal and then not be interested in food at the next. Also, if they are teething or coming down with an illness, their appetite may decrease. So don't worry too much about counting your baby's calories. Just make sure he has access to healthy sources of food, and he will let you know how much he needs.

MAKING THE SWITCH TO COW'S MILK? ─────────
The American Academy of Pediatrics recommends that for the first 12 months, babies should be fed only breast milk or iron-fortified infant formula. Cow's milk is not recommended for use in the first year of life, since cow's milk may contribute to poor iron absorption and therefore cause iron deficiency. Studies of infants who consume whole cow's milk show a significant loss of iron in stools due to an increase in intestinal blood loss. By using breast milk or iron-fortified infant formula instead, in combination with age-appropriate solid foods, you'll satisfy baby's nutritional needs. See page 45 for more on how to smoothly make the transition from breast milk to cow's milk.

What to Feed Your Toddler: A Month-by-Month Guide for 13 to 18 Months

You and baby are probably pretty used to the feeding routine, and I hope you're having a blast exploring new tastes and deciding what baby likes best. At this age, your toddler will continue to explore self-feeding, first with fingers and then with utensils. It's important to let her practice these skills, but be there to step in when she gets frustrated.

Toddlers also like to be independent at the table. Allowing them to respond to when they are hungry or full is beneficial to their development. You decide the variety of healthy foods to offer your toddler, and he can choose what and how much he wants to eat.

Refer to chapter 2 for a refresher on how much and how often you should be feeding your toddler. But in brief, you should try to offer her three meals and two or three healthy snacks a day. Don't worry if your toddler sometimes skips a meal. If you keep striving for a regular schedule of meals and snacks, your toddler will learn to expect that food will be available at certain times of day.

WHAT'S HAPPENING?

Mooooving on to Cow's Milk. At this point, most babies are transitioning from breast milk or baby formula to cow's milk. For some (especially the nursers), this process can be difficult. One of the great things about breast milk (and baby formula) is that these provide all of the nutrition baby needs; now that you are phasing them out, baby runs the risk of becoming deficient. It is important to make sure that your toddler is getting all of the nutrients that he needs, even if there is a struggle to transition away from what he has been used to drinking. Fortunately, now he can rely more on the nutrition he gets from eating the right foods.

NUTRIENT OF THE MONTH: CALCIUM

Even though 99 percent of our body's calcium is stored in our bones and teeth, it is important for so much more than just the support and function of our skeleton. Calcium is required for muscle contractions, hormone secretion, and intracellular signaling, just to name a few of its roles. For fast-growing babies and toddlers, new bone is constantly being created, hence the need for plenty of calcium. The problem is, when your baby isn't getting enough calcium, her body breaks down bone to release calcium into the blood so it can perform other necessary functions. Low calcium intake in children can lead to the development of rickets or increased risk of bone fractures later in life. Refer back to page 71, for more information on why baby needs calcium.

It isn't hard to make sure that baby gets enough calcium, a few calcium-rich food ideas include 1½ ounces cheese (about 310 mg; you can cut soft cheese into the tiniest of bits to offer baby, or shred some), 1 cup cottage cheese (about 140 mg; just avoid the store-bought kind that has fruit mixed in, as it is loaded with added sugar), or ½ cup tofu made with calcium sulfate (about 250 mg; cut into small bits). You can also try the delicious recipes that follow.

BLUEBERRY-BANANA YOGURT SMOOTHIE

MAKES 2 SERVINGS

Infinitely variable, smoothies are a fun and easy way to pack extra nutrition into breakfast or snacks. Whole-milk yogurt has calcium, vitamin B12, protein, and fat, which is important for nutrient absorption. Blueberries are a super source of vitamins K and C. The milk will give this smoothie a sweet richness that's more like a milkshake.

½ ripe banana, peeled and sliced
½ cup plain or vanilla whole-milk yogurt
½ cup frozen blueberries
½ cup milk or water

Place the banana, yogurt, blueberries, and milk into a blender and blend until smooth. Serve immediately.

SHOESTRING SWEET POTATO FRIES

MAKES 4 SERVINGS

Among potatoes, sweet potatoes have the highest amount of calcium. These baked sweet potato fries are a soft finger food that's also packed with A, B, and C vitamins. Use the dark red-skinned, orange-fleshed sweet potatoes that are commonly sold as yams.

1 pound orange-fleshed sweet potatoes (yams)
1½ tablespoons olive oil
Sea salt

Preheat the oven to 400°F.

Scrub and dry the sweet potatoes. Peel them, cut lengthwise into slices about ¼ inch thick, and then cut each slice into batons about ¼ inch wide and 3 inches long. Place on a rimmed baking sheet, drizzle on the olive oil, and toss to coat. Sprinkle lightly with salt and spread them out in an even layer. Bake, stirring with a spatula after about 10 minutes, until tender and browned on the edges, 25 minutes total. Serve immediately.

CHEESY SOFT POLENTA

MAKES 4 SERVINGS

This instant kid-comfort food cooks in just a few minutes, and it's appealing as is, with butter and cheese, or you can stir in mashed butternut squash or soft mashed pears while it's warm. Cheese adds calcium as well as other nutrients. Toddlers and older kids will enjoy it with turkey bolognese sauce (see page 130) or lamb meatballs (see page 131) spooned on top. You can slice firm polenta and reheat it in the oven with pasta sauce and cheese.

2 cups water or low-sodium chicken broth
½ cup instant polenta
¼ cup Parmesan cheese
2 teaspoons butter

In a small saucepan over medium-high heat, bring the water to a boil. Whisk in the polenta. Lower the heat to maintain a gentle simmer (it may splatter if it boils) and cook, stirring frequently, until the polenta is thick and no longer grainy, 3 to 5 minutes, or according to package instructions. Remove from the heat and stir in the cheese and butter. Let cool until just warm before serving.

To store: Polenta will set up firmly as it cools. Pour it into a shallow dish and refrigerate for up to 3 days.

WHAT'S HAPPENING?

Baby Backed Up? Now that baby is an eating machine, he is trying all different types of foods. His little tummy might not always agree with what you have on the menu, and he can get constipated. What can you do to make him feel better? Fiber is essential for baby's digestive health. (Note: See page 35 for more information on how to treat baby's constipation, and why prune juice is not the best cure.)

NUTRIENT OF THE MONTH: FIBER

While not technically a nutrient, as explained on page 72, insoluble fiber is more helpful than soluble in preventing constipation. So making sure baby gets many fruits, vegetables, and whole grains is a great way to ensure she is getting enough fiber. Processed foods (frozen meals, packaged snacks, and the like) tend to lack the fiber baby needs—all the more reason to avoid giving baby too much processed foods.

Some baby-friendly food options to boost fiber intake include 1 cup cooked lentils (15.6 g), 1 cup cooked black beans (15 g), or 1 cup cooked green peas (8.8 g). All of these are great finger or spoon foods; you can mash them up to baby's texture preference, or offer them whole for baby to try to eat on her own. In addition, try these yummy fiber-rich recipes.

FRENCH TOAST FINGERS WITH MAPLE YOGURT

MAKES 4 SERVINGS

Use any good, sturdy whole-grain bread for this sweet, handheld breakfast treat. Whole-wheat bread is a fiber- and mineral-rich carbohydrate for baby. This recipe is easily doubled so that adults and older kids can join in.

1 cup plain or vanilla Greek whole-milk yogurt
2 tablespoons maple syrup
2 eggs
⅓ cup milk
½ teaspoon ground cinnamon
1 teaspoon vanilla extract
Four ½- to ¾-inch-thick slices whole-grain bread
1 tablespoon butter

In a small bowl, mix together the yogurt and maple syrup; set aside.

In a medium bowl, whisk the eggs to blend. Gradually whisk in the milk, cinnamon, and vanilla. Pour the mixture into a shallow baking dish. Place 1 slice of bread in the milk mixture; turn over and let soak for 1 to 2 minutes.

Warm a large frying pan over medium heat. Brush the pan lightly with the butter. Add the soaked bread slice (place another slice in the mixture to soak) and cook until brown on the bottom, about 4 minutes. Turn over and cook until brown on the other side, about 4 minutes. Repeat with the remaining slices. Cut each slice into ½- to ¾-inch-wide strips.

Serve with the maple yogurt for dipping.

To store: Leftovers can be refrigerated or frozen and reheated in the toaster.

BROTHY LENTILS WITH GOAT CHEESE

MAKES 6 SERVINGS

Lentils are good to have in baby's repertoire; in addition to being a great source of fiber, they are a nutritional powerhouse. Rinse dried lentils well in a strainer, then spread them on a plate so you can see and discard any debris (like small stones) before cooking. For an even bigger fiber boost, serve with toasted whole-wheat pita wedges for dipping into the flavorful broth.

2 teaspoons olive oil
½ yellow onion, diced
1 small garlic clove, minced
1 small carrot, peeled and diced
2 cups chicken broth or water
½ cup dried brown lentils, rinsed well
One 15-ounce can crushed or pureed tomatoes
¼ teaspoon ground cumin
¼ cup crumbled fresh goat cheese

In a medium saucepan over medium heat, warm the olive oil. Add the onion, garlic, and carrot and cook, stirring frequently, until the vegetables are soft, 5 to 6 minutes.

Add the chicken broth, lentils, tomatoes, and cumin to the pan. Bring to a boil, then lower the heat to maintain a simmer. Cover and cook until the lentils are very tender, about 25 minutes. Spoon into bowls and top each with about 1 tablespoon of the goat cheese before serving.

To store: Refrigerate for up to 2 days.

RED PEPPER HUMMUS WITH STEAMED CARROT DIPPERS

MAKES 4 TO 6 SERVINGS

Toddlers love to dip! Precut and peeled "baby" carrots are an easy way for you to give them a side of fiber-rich veggies. You could also offer toasted bread or crackers for even more fiber with this baby-friendly dip; older kids and grown-ups will want to try it, too.

2 medium red bell peppers
One 15-ounce can chickpeas, strained, reserving liquid
2 tablespoons olive oil
1 teaspoon ground cumin
¼ teaspoon salt
¼ teaspoon paprika
1 tablespoon freshly squeezed lemon juice
1 cup baby carrots or carrot sticks

Preheat the oven to 450°F. Line a baking sheet with aluminum foil (to make cleanup easier).

Place the bell peppers on the baking sheet. Bake until the skins are browned and the peppers are soft, 30 to 40 minutes, turning the peppers over once midway through baking time. Set on a wire rack, cover with foil, and let steam and cool completely. Then, use a paring knife to remove the skins, seeds, and stems. (The peppers will likely come apart in pieces, which is okay.)

In a blender or food processor, whirl the chickpeas, peppers, olive oil, cumin, salt, paprika, and lemon juice until smooth. (Add water, a tablespoon at a time, as needed to make a smooth puree. Transfer the hummus to an airtight container and refrigerate for up to 3 days.)

Slice the baby carrots lengthwise into halves or quarters, depending on their thickness. Bring an inch or so of water to a boil in a pan fitted with a steamer. Place the carrots in the steamer, cover, and steam until soft, 5 to 8 minutes. Let cool completely.

Serve the hummus with the carrots for dipping.

WHAT'S HAPPENING

On the Run. By this age, most toddlers are walking. (But if yours isn't, don't worry; it sometimes takes a month or two longer.) This means he is more active than ever, and those little muscles are working overtime while he is running around exploring this new, wider world.

NUTRIENT OF THE MONTH: PROTEIN

As discussed on page 61, protein is essential for the development and maintenance of bones, muscles, and other tissues. It isn't hard to make sure baby gets enough protein, baby-friendly sources include 3 ounces meat such as ground beef (about 21 g protein; just be sure to cook it well and make the crumbles small enough for baby to handle), 1 large hard-boiled egg (6 g; you can chop it up into little pieces that baby can handle), or ½ cup cooked quinoa (4 g; great for your toddler to self-feed out of a bowl; try adding in some soft veggies, like cooked peas). If you make the quinoa with soy milk instead of water, baby gets 8 g protein! Also, try ½ cup pureed or very soft beans (about 8 g), or 1 cup whole milk (8 g). You can also try some of the following fun recipes.

UNFRIED RICE WITH PORK AND VEGETABLES

MAKES 6 SERVINGS

Tossing cooked rice with scrambled egg and diced cooked meat (both for protein) along with vegetables is practically dinner magic on busy weeknights. Best of all, you can customize it with your toddler's favorite vegetable of the moment—broccoli, spinach, or bok choy would all work.

1¾ cups water
1 cup long-grain rice
½ cup frozen peas
1 carrot, peeled and diced
1½ tablespoons low-sodium soy sauce
1 tablespoon freshly squeezed lime juice
1 tablespoon toasted sesame oil
1 teaspoon packed brown sugar
1 teaspoon grated or minced fresh ginger
2 teaspoons olive oil
2 eggs, lightly beaten
½ pound boned pork loin or boneless, skinless chicken
    breast, cut into ½-inch chunks

In a medium saucepan, bring the water to a boil. Add the rice, turn the heat to low, cover, and simmer until the rice is tender and the liquid is absorbed, about 20 minutes. Add the frozen peas and fluff with a fork. Cover to keep warm.

Meanwhile, bring an inch or so of water to a boil in a pan fitted with a steamer. Place the carrot in the steamer, cover, and steam until tender, 3 to 4 minutes. Add to the rice.

In a small bowl, mix together the soy sauce, lime juice, sesame oil, brown sugar, and ginger and set aside.

In a large nonstick frying pan over medium-high heat, warm 1 teaspoon of the olive oil. Add the egg and tilt the pan so that the egg spreads out in a thin layer. When the egg looks set (about 1 minute), break it into pieces with a spatula and add it to the rice.

Return the pan to high heat. Add the remaining 1 teaspoon oil, the pork, and about ½ tablespoon of the soy sauce mixture. Stir until the meat is no longer pink in the center (cut to test), 2 to 3 minutes; add to the rice along with the remaining soy sauce mixture. Mix well. Cut the pork into pieces small enough for your baby to handle before serving.

ORZO WITH TURKEY BOLOGNESE

MAKES 4 SERVINGS

This thick, rich sauce, made with ground turkey leg and thigh meat, is an easy pasta topping that is a good source of protein as well as iron and B vitamins. This recipe makes double the sauce you'll need for 8 ounces of pasta; freeze half (for another meal) for up to 3 months.

2 tablespoons olive oil
1 yellow onion, finely chopped
2 garlic cloves, minced
1 pound ground turkey leg and thigh meat
One 28-ounce can crushed or pureed tomatoes
¼ cup chicken broth
1 teaspoon dried oregano
½ teaspoon sea salt
⅛ teaspoon ground nutmeg
8 ounces dried whole-wheat orzo
⅓ cup grated Parmesan cheese

In a large heavy pot or Dutch oven over medium heat, warm the olive oil. Add the onion and lower the heat. Stir frequently until the onion is soft and golden, 6 to 8 minutes. Add the garlic and cook 1 minute more. Add the turkey and cook, using a spatula to crumble the meat as it cooks, until it's no longer pink, 6 to 7 minutes. Add the tomatoes, chicken broth, oregano, salt, and nutmeg. Bring the mixture to a gentle simmer, cover, and cook, stirring occasionally, until it's a thick sauce, 20 to 25 minutes.

In a 2- to 3-quart pot, bring about 1½ quarts of water to a boil. Add the orzo and cook until tender, 10 to 11 minutes. Drain well. Toss with about half the sauce and top with Parmesan cheese before serving.

what to feed your baby & toddler

LAMB MEATBALLS WITH CUCUMBER-YOGURT SAUCE

MAKES 12 TO 15 SMALL MEATBALLS

Lamb is not only a good source of protein but also a great way to get vitamin B2 (riboflavin), which is important for converting food to energy. These meatballs freeze well for up to 2 months (defrost as needed) and are a great party appetizer, too!

½ slice whole-wheat bread
1 tablespoon milk
½ pound ground lamb
Sea salt
¼ teaspoon cumin
¼ teaspoon cinnamon
1 egg yolk
1 cup whole-milk yogurt
⅓ cup peeled, shredded cucumber
2 fresh mint leaves, chopped

Preheat the oven to 400°F. Line a baking sheet with aluminum foil and brush lightly with oil.

In a food processor, process the bread into fine crumbs. In a large bowl, combine the bread crumbs and milk. Add the lamb, ¼ teaspoon salt, cumin, cinnamon, and egg yolk. Using your hands, gently combine the ingredients just until blended.

Scoop up rounded tablespoons of the mixture, roll it into balls, and set on the prepared baking sheet. Bake until the meatballs are browned and cooked through, 15 to 20 minutes.

In a small bowl, stir together the yogurt, cucumber, and mint and season with a pinch of salt, if desired.

Serve the yogurt sauce alongside the meatballs.

WHAT'S HAPPENING?

Terrible Twos Starting Early? Babies this age are gaining independence (and confidence) almost daily. Whether it be climbing onto the couch, sitting on the dog, or figuring out how to open that baby-locked cabinet, your little ball of energy is constantly thinking of new ways to have fun and explore. But with that comes frustration when her little body doesn't coordinate with her thoughts, and sometimes she may be irritable when Mom or Dad says "No" to something. You might even find that your toddler suddenly doesn't want to nap (because she has uncovered the shocking truth that life goes on while she is napping, and she can't bear the thought of missing anything!). What can you do to help baby stay positive and ward off the temper tantrums? Boost her niacin intake.

NUTRIENT OF THE MONTH: NIACIN

Niacin (vitamin B3) is important for many things, as discussed on page 65. But in addition to the health benefits of this B vitamin, there are also several behavioral benefits. Even a slight deficiency in niacin can lead to irritability, poor concentration, and restlessness, which, as you may know, are the hallmarks of toddler meltdowns and temper tantrums.

So be sure baby gets enough niacin with a variety of foods, such as 1 cup well-cooked, chopped portobello mushrooms (8 mg niacin; if the texture turns baby off, sneak it in with some ground beef); 1 cup peas (3 mg); or ¼ cup buckwheat (2 mg; if you aren't a regular buckwheat eater, try Buckwheat-Banana Pancakes [facing page], and you will be hooked!).

BUCKWHEAT-BANANA PANCAKES

MAKES 18 TO 20 PANCAKES

Buckwheat is a nutty-tasting, nutritious grain that is rich in niacin and magnesium. It's great in pancakes, especially these silver dollar–size ones, with gooey, sweet caramelized banana. Serve the pancakes with maple syrup and vanilla yogurt. This recipe makes enough for the whole family to enjoy.

1¼ cups all-purpose flour
¾ cup buckwheat flour
1½ teaspoons baking powder
1½ teaspoons baking soda
¼ teaspoon salt
2 eggs
2½ cups buttermilk
2 tablespoons butter, melted, plus more as needed
1 teaspoon vanilla extract
1 ripe banana, thinly sliced into rounds

In a large bowl, stir together the all-purpose flour, buckwheat flour, baking powder, baking soda, and salt. In a small bowl, whisk together the eggs, buttermilk, butter, and vanilla. Stir the egg mixture into the flour mixture until blended.

Warm a large frying pan or griddle over medium heat and brush lightly with butter. When the pan is hot, pour in about ⅛ cup of batter to form a mini pancake. Carefully add a few banana slices to the top. Continue adding batter and bananas, leaving enough space in the pan to flip the pancakes, and cook until the edges are set and the tops are bubbling, about 2 minutes.

Flip the pancakes and cook until golden brown on the other side, about 2 minutes more. Repeat with the remaining batter and banana slices. Serve immediately.

CREAMY TOMATO-RICE SOUP

MAKES 4 SERVINGS

This creamy soup is a filling, niacin- and vitamin C–rich comfort food (thanks to the tomatoes). And this is a great time to introduce tomatoes, if you haven't already, as baby's tummy is probably ready to handle their acidity.

1 tablespoon olive oil
½ cup chopped yellow onion
¼ teaspoon fresh thyme leaves or ⅛ teaspoon dried thyme
One 28-ounce can whole tomatoes, with their juices
1 cup chicken or vegetable broth or water
2 teaspoons sugar
3 tablespoons whipping cream (heavy cream)
1 cup cooked rice

In a medium saucepan over medium heat, warm the olive oil. Add the onion and thyme and then lower the heat. Cook, stirring occasionally, until the onion is very soft, 6 to 9 minutes.

Meanwhile, place the tomatoes and their juices in a blender or food processor and puree until smooth.

Add the pureed tomatoes, chicken broth, and sugar to the pan and simmer gently for 15 minutes, stirring occasionally. Remove from the heat and let cool for 5 to 10 minutes.

If you have an immersion blender, you can puree the soup right in the pan; otherwise, transfer it to a blender and process until smooth. (Take care, as hot liquids may spatter; leave the lid's center hole open for steam to escape and cover it with a dish towel). Return the soup to the pan and stir in the cream and rice before serving.

To store: Refrigerate for up to 2 days.

what to feed your baby & toddler

SWEET-AND-SOUR CHICKEN STIR-FRY

MAKES 3 OR 4 SERVINGS

Serve this quick, baby-friendly chicken stir-fry with steamed rice for a niacin-rich meal. The chicken is a great source of niacin for your toddler. And the best part is that this recipe is easily doubled to make a healthy dinner for the whole family.

1 tablespoon low-sodium soy sauce
2 tablespoons freshly squeezed lime juice
2 tablespoons honey
1 tablespoon olive oil
½ red bell pepper, diced
2 tablespoons minced shallots or red onion
1 skinless boneless chicken breast half (about 6 ounces), thinly sliced

In a small bowl, stir together the soy sauce, lime juice, and honey; set aside.

In a large frying pan over medium heat, warm ½ tablespoon of the olive oil. Add the bell pepper and shallots and cook until softened, 2 to 3 minutes. Transfer the mixture to a plate and add the remaining ½ tablespoon oil to the pan. Add the chicken and stir frequently until opaque and cooked through (cut it open to check), 3 to 5 minutes.

Return the bell pepper and shallots to the pan and stir in the soy sauce mixture. Cook just until heated through, about 1 minute. Cut the chicken into small pieces before feeding baby.

To store: Refrigerate for up to 2 days.

WHAT'S HAPPENING?

It Takes Guts to Be a Toddler. It really does take a lot of guts to do all of the brave things your little one does, from trying new foods to making new friends. In addition to those mental-emotional guts, babies this age also need to have good digestive health to avoid diaper rash issues or tummy pains.

NUTRIENT OF THE MONTH: FOLATE

As discussed on pages 66 to 67, folate is necessary to create healthy red blood cells, which are important for promoting your toddler's digestive health. Your baby can get 50 percent of her folate requirements with only one-fourth of a very ripe cantaloupe, well diced. (If you think the fruit is too hard, puree it and pour it into a cup for baby to drink.) Other sources include 5 spears asparagus (100 mcg folate; you can steam and puree them and add to rice or mix with other pureed veggies to make baby a "soup"), 8 strawberries (80 mcg; just make sure they are either cut small enough or pureed to prevent choking), or 2 tablespoons smooth peanut butter (25 mcg; try swirling it into fortified oatmeal). In addition, try some of the following recipes. Now that baby is getting bigger, you can start doubling the batches, and baby can share these with you (or make even more for the rest of the family).

PAPAYA-KIWI-STRAWBERRY SALSA

MAKES ABOUT 1½ CUPS

Little cubes of bright fresh fruit are a folate and vitamin C bonanza!
Serve this alongside a quesadilla (try Smashed Pinto Bean Quesadillas,
below), on top of yogurt, or by itself.

½ small papaya, peeled, seeded, and diced
½ kiwi, peeled and diced
½ cup diced strawberries

Combine the fruit in a bowl and mix well before serving.

To store: Refrigerate for up to 1 day.

SMASHED PINTO BEAN QUESADILLAS

MAKES 2 SERVINGS

Quesadillas are a fast and easy toddler favorite. Baby gets a great boost
of folate from the avocado and beans in this delicious dish.

½ ripe avocado, pitted and coarsely mashed
Two 8-inch whole-wheat flour tortillas
¼ cup canned refried pinto beans or drained cooked pinto beans,
    lightly mashed
¼ cup shredded Monterey Jack cheese
1 teaspoon olive oil
Sour cream and salsa for serving (optional; but pairs well with
    Papaya-Kiwi-Strawberry Salsa, above)

Spread the avocado evenly over one tortilla; top with the beans, cheese,
and second tortilla. Lightly brush the top tortilla with about ½ teaspoon
of the olive oil.

In a pan over medium heat, warm the remaining ½ teaspoon olive oil.
Place the quesadilla in the pan (unoiled-side down) and cook until lightly
browned on the bottom, 1 to 2 minutes. Turn it over gently with a wide
spatula (or, to keep the filling neatly inside, transfer to a cutting board,
top with another board, grasp the "sandwich" firmly and turn over, then
slide the flipped quesadilla back into the pan, cooked-side up). Cook the
other side until the bottom is lightly browned and the cheese is melted.
Cut into eight wedges to serve.

FALAFEL SLIDERS

MAKES 6 SLIDERS

These little patties are packed with folate, thanks to the chickpeas, and have a nice green hit of vitamin C, too. Mix up an optional tahini-yogurt sauce by blending ½ cup plain yogurt, 1 tablespoon tahini (sesame paste), and 1 tablespoon freshly squeezed lemon juice, then season with salt. If tahini sauce isn't to your toddler's taste, there's no reason you can't put ketchup on these savory little burgers, since they offer many other nutrients.

1½ cups canned or cooked dried chickpeas
1 egg yolk
¼ cup minced red onion
2 garlic cloves, peeled
1 cup fresh parsley leaves
1 tablespoon freshly squeezed lemon juice
2 teaspoons Dijon mustard
2 tablespoons all-purpose flour
2 tablespoons white sesame seeds
1 teaspoon baking powder
1 teaspoon ground cumin
½ teaspoon salt
2 tablespoons olive oil
6 mini pitas or slider buns

In a blender or food processor, combine the chickpeas, egg yolk, onion, garlic, parsley, lemon juice, and mustard. Pulse until the mixture forms a coarse paste. Transfer to a bowl and stir in the flour, sesame seeds, baking powder, cumin, and salt. Chill until cold, about 1 hour or up to 1 day.

In a large nonstick skillet over medium-high heat, warm 1 tablespoon of the olive oil. With wet hands, form about ¼ cup of the mixture into a ½-inch-thick patty. Add to the pan and repeat with the remaining mixture, in two batches if necessary. Cook until the patties are crisp and browned, 2 to 3 minutes on each side.

Place the patties in mini pitas or on slider buns; cut into pieces your toddler can handle before serving.

To store: Cooled patties freeze well and can be reheated in the oven for a fast lunch or dinner. Place wax paper between them and seal in a ziplock plastic bag; freeze for up to 2 months.

what to feed your baby & toddler

WHAT'S HAPPENING?

Make a Mental Note: Your toddler is about to cross into being closer to age 2 than to age 1. She is growing fast, and her little brain is working hard all day long to master new things. She is continually learning to make associations, grasp the meanings of words, and effectively communicate with you. All that takes brain power, and brains run on neurotransmitters!

NUTRIENT OF THE MONTH: VITAMIN B6

Vitamin B6 is important for a lot of things (flip back to page 66, if you need a refresher), but mainly it is essential for brain health and making neurotransmitters. It is easy to boost brain power with plenty of vitamin B6. A few baby-friendly ideas on how you can ramp up vitamin B6 intake include 1 medium banana (0.4 mg vitamin B6; don't cut it in circular slices, as baby can choke, try strips or wedges); 1 ounce hazelnuts (0.2 mg; baby will love it if you puree them to make your own nut butter and add it to cooked cereal, or a spread on a slice of bread that you then cut into strips); ½ cup diced pitted prunes (0.2 mg); 1 cup mashed sweet potato (0.3 mg); 1 cup cooked, canned chickpeas (1.1 mg; a great finger food); or 1 cup boiled and mashed potatoes (0.4 mg). In addition, check out the vitamin B6–rich recipes that follow.

LOADED SWEET POTATO SKINS

MAKES 4 SERVINGS

These crispy sweet potato skins are an irresistible snack for adults and older kids, too, and provide a good dose of the vitamin B6 that your toddler needs. Choose organic sweet potatoes, since you're eating the skins, and scrub them well. This recipe makes enough for you to enjoy with baby.

2 small dark red-skinned sweet potatoes (yams)
Olive oil for rubbing
Salt and freshly ground black pepper
¼ to ⅓ cup cooked, drained black beans, partially mashed,
    or canned refried black beans
½ cup shredded cheddar cheese
3 tablespoons plain Greek yogurt
2 tablespoons minced green onions (optional)
¼ cup tomato salsa (optional)

Preheat the oven to 400°F.

Scrub the sweet potatoes well. Prick several holes in each potato with a skewer or paring knife and rub the skins lightly with olive oil. Place them on a baking sheet. Bake until the potatoes are soft when you pierce them with a knife, 40 to 50 minutes.

Let the potatoes cool until you can handle them comfortably and then cut each in half lengthwise. Scoop out the center, leaving about ½ inch thickness of flesh attached to the skin. (Save the scooped-out flesh for another use.)

Sprinkle each half lightly with salt and pepper and top with about 1 tablespoon of the beans and 1 to 2 tablespoons of the cheese. Place the loaded skins on the baking sheet and place under the broiler or return to the oven until the cheese is melted and the edges are crisp, 1 to 2 minutes.

Let cool and top each with a dollop of yogurt and the green onions and salsa, if desired. Cut into small pieces your toddler can handle before serving.

CARROT COINS WITH HONEY BUTTER

MAKES 1 SERVING

These cheerful rounds may become your go-to side dish, and the carrots can help meet your toddler's vitamin B6 needs. It's easy to make just as much as you need.

2 small carrots, peeled and cut into ¼-inch rounds
½ tablespoon butter
2 teaspoons honey
Pinch of salt

Bring several inches of water to boil in a pan fitted with a steamer. Place the carrots in the steamer, cover, and steam until they are very soft when you pierce them with a knife, 6 to 8 minutes. Transfer to a bowl.

In a small saucepan (or a small bowl in the microwave), melt the butter and honey together with the salt. Stir and drizzle over the carrots; mix to coat. Mash slightly or cut into small pieces before serving baby.

To store: Cover and refrigerate for up to 1 day.

MINI BROCCOLI FRITTATAS

MAKES 12 FRITTATAS

Broccoli for breakfast? For sure. Baby gets vitamin B6 from the broccoli, eggs, and milk. Make a batch of these little egg muffins—they keep in the refrigerator for up to 3 days—and then reheat them individually in the microwave for breakfast, lunch, or snacks. (Don't worry; despite the rumors, nuking your food won't destroy the nutrients.)

Olive oil for brushing (optional)
½ pound broccoli florets
10 eggs
½ cup grated sharp cheddar cheese
⅓ cup milk
¼ teaspoon salt

Preheat the oven to 350°F. Brush the insides of a 12-cup muffin tin generously with olive oil or line with paper liners.

Bring several inches of water to boil in a pan fitted with a steamer. Place the broccoli in the steamer, cover, and steam until tender, 5 to 6 minutes. Let cool and then roughly chop.

In a large bowl, lightly whisk the eggs, cheese, milk, and salt until blended.

Divide the broccoli evenly among the prepared muffin cups. Using a measuring cup, pour about ¼ cup of the egg mixture into each cup, covering the broccoli.

Bake until the frittatas are puffy, browned, and set in the center, 18 to 20 minutes. Let cool in the pan for 5 minutes, then loosen the edges with a knife and gently remove. Serve warm or at room temperature.

***

Your baby is growing like a weed, thanks to the nutritious foods that you are preparing for him each day. In this chapter, we've covered the key nutrients and corresponding foods that are good for your toddler to consume once he has graduated from pureed to finger foods. In the next chapter, we will discuss some ways you can keep your self-feeder eating well, while he is taking bigger bites.

Sample Menus for Ages 13 to 18 Months

These sample menus can give you some ideas for how to combine foods for baby. Feel free to mix and match to baby's preference.

ONE-DAY SAMPLE MENU—13 TO 18 MONTHS	
Breakfast	French Toast Fingers with Maple Yogurt (page 125) ¼ cup whole milk 1 small banana, sliced
Snack	½ cup iron-fortified cereal ¼ cup raspberries ½ cup whole milk
Lunch	2 ounces cooked ground beef ½ cup cooked broccoli ¼ cup brown rice or Unfried Rice with Pork and Vegetables (page 129)
Snack	1 slice whole-wheat toast, cut up Red Pepper Hummus with Steamed Carrot Dippers (page 127)
Dinner	Brothy Lentils with Goat Cheese (page 126) ¼ cup well-cooked, chopped green beans ½ cup whole milk

ONE-DAY SAMPLE MENU—13 TO 18 MONTHS	
Breakfast	½ cup iron-fortified breakfast cereal Blueberry-Banana Yogurt Smoothie (page 122)
Snack	1 to 2 ounces string cheese (diced) ¼ cup raspberries
Lunch	2 ounces cod baked with olive oil Cheesy Soft Polenta (page 123) ⅓ cup well-cooked, chopped asparagus
Snack	1 ounce whole-wheat pita slices 2 tablespoons mashed white beans ½ cup whole milk
Dinner	¼ cup whole-wheat pasta, well cooked ⅓ to ½ cup well-cooked, chopped beets Mini Broccoli Frittatas (facing page)

6

Bigger Bites (19 to 24 Months)

Can you believe how quickly your toddler is growing? So much is happening with your little one these days that you are likely to be exhausted trying to keep up.

This chapter will cover the basics on feeding your toddler from ages 19 to 24 months. By now, you have a fully functioning independent feeder, who most likely won't let you put a spoon with a puree on it anywhere near him! Your toddler is the boss and likely has his favorite (and not-so-favorite) foods. Also, he most likely exercises his right to change his mind quite often, and you will probably see that certain foods are happily eaten one day and scoffed at the next. That's okay. It doesn't mean your toddler will turn up his nose at them forever, but it does mean that your baby is maturing enough so that you may want to limit the number of options at mealtimes—otherwise, you will let him turn you into a short-order cook.

Like the previous two chapters, this one will briefly cover what is happening with your toddler developmentally during this time and then focus on a nutrient of the month that is key to baby's health and development. It will also give you a list of foods high in that nutrient to help you make sure your toddler is getting what she needs to keep growing healthy and strong. In addition, more recipes are provided for each month; and now that your toddler can handle bigger bites, these recipes can be made for the whole family to enjoy.

Remember, I go over the nitty-gritty of how much baby needs (in terms of calorie and nutrition requirements) in chapters 2 and 3 and offer advice and tips on making feeding baby fun. So be sure to review if you need a refresher.

What's Happening Developmentally? An Overview

As your baby approaches age 2, a lot is happening. Physically, you may have noticed that his growth has slowed a bit. While he is still growing, it isn't quite as rapid as it was up until this point. So go ahead and invest in some nice 2T clothes; your toddler will get a few more wearings out of them than he did with his infant clothes.

Emotionally, around this age, many toddlers start to become more accepting of new people. If your little one is still shy, that is okay. Some people just have that personality from an early age, and it may take her longer to warm up to strangers.

Cognitively, your toddler probably likes to show off how independent she is. From picking out her own clothes to having a favorite toy or doll, she likely knows what she wants (and doesn't want). Language continues to develop, and you will notice her probably starting to put words together. Each day, she is making new associations and learning the meaning of the words you use, so be sure to point things out to her as much as you can. At this early learning age, toddlers also make some very cute (and understandable) word association errors. For example, if your little one calls the dog "woof," she might also say "woof" when she sees other four-legged creatures, such as horses. This is a good sign that she is thinking about what the words she uses actually mean.

Getting Started

Bigger toddlers can have bigger bites, meaning that they can have slightly larger pieces of food because they have more teeth and better control. But still be mindful of choking and use proper supervision. While they have more teeth, they still need to chew their food thoroughly to make sure they swallow it without incident. Also, an added challenge that you may not have faced as much up until this point is that 2-year-olds are busy people, and they don't always want to sit down for a meal. But your toddler does need to stay put while he eats.

As your toddler matures and becomes more independent, you may find that it is difficult to get him to eat foods that he may have loved in the past. You may have to offer him a choice, to some extent, and allow him to make decisions about what he will eat. That doesn't mean letting him dictate the menu each day. Offer small portions of two or three healthy options, and he can pick what he wants to eat. Like many adults, toddlers are more likely to cooperate with a plan when they have some say in it.

FOOD FOR THOUGHT If you think about it, you might actually benefit from following your baby's diet guidelines. By preparing all your family's food in a baby-friendly way, without too much added salt and using as few processed foods as possible, you may find your own diet improving. Considering that your child is going to quickly start copying and modeling her behavior after yours, especially when it comes to eating, why not take advantage of this opportunity to fine-tune your own diet?

What to Feed Your Toddler: A Month-by-Month Guide for 19 to 24 Months

By this point, your toddler has had the opportunity to explore many different tastes and textures, and can feed himself relatively independently. But remember that baby should always be supervised when eating, as you want to not only make sure he stays safe but also encourage good manners. At this age, your toddler will still probably prefer to use his fingers, but now is a great time to encourage him to eat with utensils. His hand-eye coordination continues to get better, so he can handle a fork and spoon.

Refer back to pages 23 and 28 for a reminder on how much and how often you should be feeding your toddler. In general, you should continue to try to offer your child three meals and two or three healthful snacks a day, but it is still okay if your toddler skips snacks or meals once in a while. Also, at this age, many children are well aware of the concept of "dessert," so don't forget to have some healthy treats on hand so that your little one can indulge without too much added sugar.

WHAT'S HAPPENING?

Running on Fumes? You might feel like you are in need of an IV drip of coffee to get through the day chasing after your 19-month-old. Babies this age are into everything. If they aren't asking for you to play with them, get them a drink, get them a snack, and get them crayons (all within the span of 3 minutes!), they are pulling out every toy you own and trashing the room the minute you turn your back. All this work can make you (and baby) weak with exhaustion.

NUTRIENT OF THE MONTH: POTASSIUM

While the job of being a toddler is enough to drain anyone, baby also might become sluggish if he is low in potassium, as this can lead to weakness and fatigue. High-potassium foods will help give him the energy he needs to go all day (and then, you hope, sleep all night).

In addition to the ideas for increasing potassium intake mentioned on page 75, you can try these baby-friendly foods to boost potassium levels: 1 cup cooked acorn squash (900 mg potassium; dice small or puree), ½ cup dried apricots (about 750 mg; cook and dice small), 1 cup kidney beans (715 mg; cook well and mash), 1 cup yogurt (580 mg), 1 cup chopped zucchini (450 mg), or 1 veggie burger (250 mg; crumble into baby-friendly bits). Also, check out the following yummy recipes that not only will boost potassium levels for baby but also are high in fiber.

OATMEAL APPLESAUCE MUFFINS

MAKES 12 MUFFINS

These are like apple-cinnamon oatmeal baked into a hearty handheld breakfast or snack. Baby gets added potassium from the applesauce and oats.

1½ cups whole-wheat flour
¾ cup rolled oats
2 teaspoons baking powder
½ teaspoon baking soda
¾ teaspoon cinnamon
½ teaspoon salt
1 cup applesauce (opt for the "no added sugar" variety)
⅔ cup packed dark or light brown sugar
⅓ cup olive or canola oil
1 egg

Preheat the oven to 350°F. Line a 12-cup muffin tin with paper liners.

In a medium bowl, stir together the flour, oats, baking powder, baking soda, cinnamon, and salt. In a large bowl, whisk together the applesauce, brown sugar, olive oil, and egg until well blended. Stir in the flour mixture until mostly combined, with a few remaining lumps; avoid overmixing. Divide the batter evenly among the muffin cups.

Bake until the tops are set and golden brown, 25 to 30 minutes. Let cool for 5 minutes in the pan, then gently remove the muffins and set on a baking rack to cool completely before serving.

To store: Transfer to an airtight container at room temperature for up to 1 day, or freeze for up to 1 month.

MEDJOOL DATE–ORANGE SALAD

Sweet orange segments and soft, fresh, potassium-packed dates make a sweet-tangy salad. In citrus season, try Cara Cara oranges, sometimes called pink navel oranges.

1 orange
2 fresh Medjool dates

With a sharp knife, cut off and discard the ends of the orange. Stand the orange on one flat end on a cutting board. Using the knife and following the curve of the fruit, carefully slice off the peel and outer membrane. Cut in between the segments and the inner membranes to release the fruit. (Discard the membranes.) Cut each segment into bite-size pieces. Halve and pit the dates and dice into small cubes. In a medium bowl, gently combine the fruits. Serve immediately.

STICKY RICE BALLS WITH SALMON

MAKES 6 RICE BALLS

Make this fun finger food when you have a little bit of cooked salmon left over; it delivers a nice boost of potassium. Older kids will like helping shape these delicious rice balls, called *onigiri* in Japan, where they are a favorite lunch or snack. A rice cooker is an easy, mess-free, and reliable way to cook rice, so if you have one, do use it.

¾ cup short-grain (sushi) rice
1¼ cups water, plus more as needed
2 teaspoons rice vinegar
About ¼ cup flaked cooked salmon
Soy sauce for dipping

Rinse the rice. In a medium saucepan, bring the water to a boil. Add the rice, turn the heat to low, cover, and simmer until the rice is tender and the water is absorbed, about 20 minutes. Let stand, covered, for 5 minutes. Stir in 1 teaspoon of the vinegar and let cool to warm room temperature.

Place a sheet of wax paper on your work surface. Fill a small bowl with about ½ cup cold water and add the remaining 1 teaspoon vinegar. Wet your hands in the vinegar water. Place about ¼ cup rice on your work surface and use your wet hands to pat it into a 4-inch round. Place a small piece of salmon in the center and form the rice into a ball around it. (If the rice sticks to your hands, wet your hands again.)

Rice balls are best eaten at room temperature within a few hours. Serve with soy sauce for dipping.

WHAT'S HAPPENING?

Yak, Yak, Yak. Remember back when you wished baby would talk and fretted over whether she would ever speak? Perhaps you are longing for those days, now that your little motormouth won't let you get a word into the conversation!

NUTRIENT OF THE MONTH: MANGANESE

As mentioned on pages 74 to 75, manganese is needed for baby's brain to function properly. And you need to have a healthy brain for language development to occur. Serving foods rich in manganese is a great way to make sure baby stays on track in the speech department. Some good sources of manganese for baby are ½ cup pineapple (0.77 mg; chop into baby-size pieces), ½ cup brown rice (1.07 mg), or ½ cup mashed sweet potatoes (0.44 mg).

In addition to the sources mentioned in chapter 3, you can also try these great recipes, which feature foods rich in mangsanese.

SESAME SOBA NOODLES WITH ASPARAGUS

MAKES 4 SERVINGS

Soba is a Japanese noodle made with buckwheat, a nutty-tasting grain that is a nutritious alternative to pasta. Soba noodles are susceptible to overcooking, so keep them on the al dente side. As an added bonus, the asparagus in this dish gives baby a nice dose of manganese. This makes enough for dinner for everyone, and any leftovers can be enjoyed cold by baby (and you!) the next day.

¾ pound slender asparagus
3 tablespoons toasted sesame oil
2 tablespoons low-sodium soy sauce
1½ tablespoons freshly squeezed lemon juice
2 teaspoons tahini
8 ounces dried soba noodles, broken in half
1 tablespoon olive oil
1 tablespoon grated or minced fresh ginger
1 garlic clove, pressed or minced

Trim the stem ends of the asparagus. Cut each spear in half lengthwise. Cut each length into ½-inch pieces.

In a small bowl, stir together the sesame oil, soy sauce, lemon juice, and tahini until smooth. Set aside.

Bring a large pot of water to a boil. Add the soba noodles and cook gently, stirring once or twice, for 3 minutes. Add the asparagus to the water and boil until the noodles and asparagus are tender, about 3 minutes more. Drain, then rinse the noodles and asparagus briefly under cold running water to keep the noodles from sticking together.

In a large frying pan over medium-high heat, warm the olive oil. Add the ginger and garlic and cook until fragrant, about 1 minute. Add the noodles, asparagus, and sesame oil mixture to the pan and stir until the noodles are well coated, about 2 minutes. Serve immediately.

HERBED BROWN BASMATI RICE

MAKES 4 SERVINGS

If your family includes cilantro fans, now's a good time to find out if baby is among the approximately 10 percent of humans who experience a chemical revulsion to the herb. (Note: If either Mom or Dad find cilantro to taste soapy, that ups the odds; these odor receptors appear to be genetic.) If she is, just use basil or parsley instead. Brown rice is a good source of not only fiber but also important minerals, including manganese, selenium, copper, and magnesium. This is an easy side dish for a toddler who is ready to eat with the grown-ups—it goes wonderfully with Marinated Grilled Chicken Kabobs (page 156).

¾ cup brown basmati rice
Pinch of salt
1½ cups water
½ tablespoon butter
1 teaspoon chopped fresh cilantro, basil, or parsley

In a medium saucepan, combine the rice, salt, and water and bring to a boil over medium-high heat (or use rice cooker if you have one). Turn the heat to low, cover, and simmer until the liquid is absorbed and the rice is tender, 20 to 25 minutes. Fluff the rice with a fork and mix in the butter and chopped herbs before serving.

ALMOND BUTTER AND RASPBERRY JAM PINWHEELS

MAKES 6 PIECES

This fast sandwich is a vehicle for nutritious nut and seed butters of all kinds. Almond butter is great because it boasts a nice amount of manganese for baby's brain health. Other combos to try are cashew butter with apricot jam, peanut butter with honey, and sunflower seed butter with strawberry jam.

1 whole-wheat tortilla
2 tablespoons almond butter
1½ to 2 tablespoons low- or no-sugar raspberry preserves

Spread the tortilla with the almond butter and jam, and roll it tightly. Slice into 1-inch rounds to serve.

WHAT'S HAPPENING?

AHHHH-CHOOOO! Babies get sick. It's a fact of life. At this age, your toddler may be exposed to even more people than before, in playgroups, music groups, or day care. But you can help baby be better able to fight off infections by making sure he's getting the right balance of nutrients.

NUTRIENT OF THE MONTH: SELENIUM

As discussed on page 76, selenium is needed for your baby's thyroid to function normally, and it plays important roles in DNA synthesis and preventing infection. Selenium also protects cells from oxidative damage and is needed for optimum bone health as well as blood-sugar control. Making sure your toddler gets enough selenium is a great way to ward off those nasty infections that little ones tend to pick up. One of the best sources of selenium is Brazil nuts, but make sure to grind them up since they can be a choking hazard (6 to 8 nuts have around 544 mcg). Many varieties of seafood are excellent sources of selenium, including 3 ounces halibut (47 mcg) and 3 ounces sardines (45 mcg), as well as meats, such as 3 ounces ground beef (33 mcg) and 3 ounces ground turkey (31 mcg). One cup of cottage cheese provides 20 mcg of selenium.

In addition to the great ways in which you can use food to boost baby's selenium intake that I noted in chapter 3, try the following recipes. They are loaded with not only selenium but other important nutrients to help keep baby healthy and strong.

MARINATED GRILLED CHICKEN KABOBS

MAKES 4 SKEWERS

These mildly spiced, toddler-friendly kabobs go great with Herbed Brown Basmati Rice (page 154). Serve additional yogurt on the side if you like. This dish provides baby with many nutrients, including selenium from the yogurt, ginger, and chicken. You will need to soak four wooden skewers in water while the chicken is marinating.

¾ cup plain whole-milk yogurt
Freshly squeezed juice of ½ lemon
1 garlic clove, minced
1 teaspoon grated or minced ginger
2 tablespoons paprika
1 teaspoon ground cumin
1 teaspoon ground coriander
½ teaspoon salt
½- to ¾-pound boneless, skinned chicken breast half,
    cut into 1½-inch chunks

Preheat a grill to medium-hot and oil it.

In a bowl large enough to hold the chicken, mix the yogurt with the lemon juice, garlic, ginger, paprika, cumin, coriander, and salt. Add the chicken pieces and stir to coat. Cover and refrigerate for 30 minutes.

Thread the chicken pieces equally onto four water-soaked wooden skewers. Grill the chicken, turning once, until cooked through, 7 to 9 minutes total.

Push the chicken off the skewers and let cool. Cut it into small pieces your toddler can handle, and serve.

To store: Refrigerate for up to 2 days.

CHICKEN NOODLE EGG-DROP SOUP
WITH BABY BOK CHOY

MAKES 4 SERVINGS

This is a super-fast selenium-rich dinner to make if you have cooked chicken and veggies on hand. Other vegetables would be great in this soup too; just be sure to dice them into small pieces and cook them until tender. This recipe makes enough for you to enjoy with baby.

½ cup small dried pasta shapes, such as alphabet letters, orzo, or stars
1 egg
4 ounces baby bok choy
3½ cups homemade or low-sodium chicken broth
1 cup diced cooked chicken
1 teaspoon soy sauce

Bring a medium saucepan of water to a boil over high heat. Add the pasta and cook until tender, according to package directions. Drain.

In a small bowl, scramble the egg with 1 teaspoon water.

Separate the bok choy leaves, rinse them well, and chop finely.

In a medium saucepan over medium heat, bring the chicken broth to a boil. Add the bok choy and simmer until tender, 4 to 5 minutes.

Add the chicken and cooked pasta to the pan and bring the soup to a simmer. Pour in the egg and stir gently until the egg is set, about 1 minute. Stir in the soy sauce before serving.

QUICK TURKEY CHILI

MAKES 4 SERVINGS

Ground turkey and pinto beans make a protein- and iron-packed dish that also has selenium. This mildly spiced chili can be served with grated cheese on top or rolled up in a tortilla.

1 tablespoon olive oil
½ cup diced yellow onion
1 garlic clove, pressed or minced
1 pound ground turkey leg and/or thigh meat
1 tablespoon mild chili powder
½ teaspoon ground cumin
¼ teaspoon dried oregano
¼ teaspoon sea salt
One 15-ounce can crushed tomatoes
1½ cups cooked or canned pinto beans
½ cup shredded cheddar cheese

In a medium saucepan over medium heat, warm the olive oil. Add the onion and lower the heat. Cook, stirring frequently, until the onion is soft and golden, 5 to 6 minutes. Add the garlic and cook 1 to 2 minutes more.

Add the turkey, chili powder, cumin, oregano, and salt to the pan and stir, crumbling the turkey with a spatula as it cooks, until the meat is no longer pink, about 5 minutes. Add the tomatoes and beans and bring to a simmer. Turn the heat to low, cover, and simmer gently for 15 minutes. Spoon into bowls and top with the cheese to serve.

To store: Refrigerate for up to 3 days or freeze for up to 3 months.

WHAT'S HAPPENING?

Boo-Boo. You may find that your most frequently used word these days is "Walk!!" Toddlers this age typically move at one of two speeds: fast or faster. Your toddler has a lot to do, and running from place to place is the most efficient way for him to get around. This means, of course, that he is bound to have some falls, and sometimes he can cut or scrape himself in the process. What can you do to make sure baby's boo-boos heal quickly? Boost his vitamin K intake.

NUTRIENT OF THE MONTH: VITAMIN K

On page 70, I note the importance of vitamin K in a balanced diet; one body function it helps with is clotting. Without the proper level of vitamin K, your toddler may bleed or bruise easily. Foods rich in vitamin K to try are ½ cup collard greens (530 mcg vitamin K; try these sautéed in a little oil and pureed, and added to another dish), 1 cup raw kale (113 mcg; raw kale is likely too fibrous for your baby to chew, so try it sautéed in oil and then pureed and added to a dish), ½ cup edamame (21 mcg; steamed well, makes a great finger food), or 1 ounce pureed cashews (10 mcg; process until smooth to make your own nut butter, which you can spread on pita bread and then cut into fun shapes). In addition, try the following recipes.

WAFFLE PANINI WITH CREAM CHEESE AND FRUIT PRESERVES

MAKES 1 SANDWICH

Enlist your kitchen gadgets to do double duty and use your waffle iron to make fun pressed sandwiches—toddlers will like the bumpy pattern it creates on the bread! Almond butter, honey, and bananas make another good waffle-sandwich filling. And baby won't know it, but this is a great source of vitamin K, thanks to the bread and butter!

1½ tablespoons softened cream cheese
Two 2½-inch-thick slices soft bread, such as challah
1½ tablespoons low- or no-sugar fruit jam
Butter for grilling

Heat the waffle iron. Spread the cream cheese on one slice of bread and the jam on the other. Close the sandwich, lightly butter the outsides, and place in the waffle iron until crisp and golden, 3 to 4 minutes. Let cool completely and then cut the sandwich into strips your toddler can handle before serving.

CHICKEN-MANGO SALAD MINI PITAS

MAKES 6 SANDWICHES

This toddler-friendly chicken salad is high in vitamin K and tangy and fresh-tasting, thanks to the lime juice and Greek yogurt. It makes a great picnic sandwich! For grown-ups, feel free to mix in some diced red onion and a little Dijon mustard after you've set aside a portion for your toddler. Refrigerate leftover chicken salad for up to 1 day.

½ cup plain whole-milk Greek yogurt
Freshly squeezed juice of 1 lime
Pinch of salt
2 cups finely diced cooked chicken
1 large ripe mango, peeled, pitted, and diced
½ red bell pepper, seeded and minced
6 mini pita rounds, split

In a bowl, whisk together the yogurt, lime juice, and salt. Add the chicken, mango, and bell pepper and stir to combine. Spoon into the pita rounds to serve.

GREEN RISOTTO

MAKES 4 SERVINGS

This is a shortcut, creamy risotto-like dish that's packed with spinach (and vitamin K) and is extra kid-friendly. Pass additional Parmesan on the side! This recipe yields plenty for you to enjoy with your baby.

2 cups packed washed baby spinach leaves
1 cup arborio rice
3 to 3½ cups chicken, beef, or vegetable broth
1 tablespoon olive oil or butter
¼ cup grated Parmesan cheese
Sea salt

Place the spinach in a steamer and set in a saucepan with an inch or so of water in the bottom. Cover tightly, bring the water to a boil, and steam until the spinach is bright green and wilted, 1 to 2 minutes.

Transfer the spinach to a food processor. Puree until smooth, stopping to scrape the sides of the bowl a few times and adding a little water if necessary to get the right consistency.

In a small saucepan over medium-high heat, combine the rice and 3 cups of the broth and bring to a boil. Turn the heat to low, cover, and cook, stirring frequently, until the liquid is absorbed and the rice is soft and creamy, about 20 minutes. If you want a softer consistency, add another ¼ cup broth and continue to cook for several minutes longer. Let cool for 10 minutes, then stir in the olive oil and Parmesan cheese and season with salt. Stir in the spinach and thin with the remaining ¼ cup broth, if desired, before serving.

WHAT'S HAPPENING?

First Haircut. Even if you had a bald little baby, by now your toddler probably has a full head of lovely locks. You may even need to start getting it cut regularly. Having healthy hair and skin isn't just a concern for us adults!

NUTRIENT OF THE MONTH: VITAMIN B1

As explained on page 64, vitamin B1 (also called thiamine) is essential for the process of converting food into energy, and it is also necessary for healthy skin, hair, and heart. The right nutrient balance can help keep baby's hair healthy and her skin clear and soft. Remember, the skin (including the scalp) is an organ. It is important that we care for it, just as we take care of our heart and lungs. Using sunscreen and wearing a hat is a must for your toddler, and so is eating healthful foods.

A few baby-friendly ideas for ways you can boost vitamin B1 levels include 1 ounce shredded lean pork (0.3 mg thiamine) or 1 slice whole-wheat bread (0.14 mg) smeared with ⅓ avocado (0.34 mg). Also check out these vitamin B1–packed recipes.

QUICK SPINACH-POTATO SOUP

MAKES ABOUT 2 CUPS

There are good reasons to include spinach in your toddler's diet whenever you can—it's a great source of critical minerals and vitamins, including B1, K, A, folate, and iron. Adults may discover that adding a little olive oil, salt, and Parmesan cheese to this combo yields a new favorite lunch recipe.

1 medium russet potato
1 cup tightly packed washed baby spinach leaves
1 to 1½ cups chicken or vegetable broth
Salt
Olive oil for drizzling
Grated Parmesan cheese for sprinkling (optional)

Rinse and peel the potato and cut into 1-inch chunks. Bring several inches of water to boil in a pan fitted with a steamer. Place the potato in the steamer, cover, and steam until the potato is very soft when you pierce it with a knife, 8 to 10 minutes. Add the spinach leaves to the steamer, cover, and steam until the spinach is bright green and wilted, 1 to 2 minutes more. Let cool.

Transfer the potato and spinach to a blender with 1 cup of the broth and process until smooth. Add the remaining ½ cup broth as needed to get the right consistency. Pour into a saucepan and reheat gently. Season with salt, drizzle with olive oil, and sprinkle with Parmesan cheese, if desired, before serving.

To store: Refrigerate for up to 2 days or freeze individual portions for up to 3 months.

APRICOT-OAT SQUARES

MAKES 16 SQUARES

Dried apricots are a sweet and tasty source of vitamin B1, iron, fiber, and potassium. You can make the dough for these fruit-filled cookies several days ahead and store it in the refrigerator. The dried fruit filling is easiest to spread the day you make the squares.

FOR THE CRUST
½ cup unsalted butter, softened
⅔ cup packed light brown sugar
1 egg
1 teaspoon vanilla
1½ cups all-purpose flour
½ cup rolled oats
1 teaspoon baking powder
¼ teaspoon salt

FOR THE FILLING
½ cup water, plus more as needed
2 tablespoons granulated sugar
Pinch of salt
2 teaspoons freshly squeezed lemon juice
8 ounces dried apricot halves, roughly chopped
½ teaspoon vanilla

TO MAKE THE CRUST Line an 8-inch-square baking pan with aluminum foil, leaving a little overhang.

In a medium bowl, beat together the butter and brown sugar until smooth and creamy. Beat in the egg and vanilla until well blended. In a small bowl, mix together the flour, oats, baking powder, and salt.

Stir the flour mixture into the butter mixture until well blended. Divide the dough in half and pat one half evenly into the bottom of the prepared pan. Wrap the other half of dough in plastic and place the pan and wrapped dough in the refrigerator to chill until firm, at least 1 hour or up to 1 day.

what to feed your baby & toddler

TO MAKE THE FILLING In a small saucepan over medium heat, combine the water, granulated sugar, salt, and lemon juice and stir until the sugar is dissolved and the mixture comes to a boil. Add the apricots and vanilla and remove from the heat. Cover and let stand at room temperature until cool, about 30 minutes. Puree the mixture (including any unabsorbed liquid) in a food processor until smooth. Add additional water, 1 tablespoon at a time, if needed to make a thick, smooth paste. Scrape into a bowl, cover, and set aside.

Preheat oven to 375°F.

Spread the cooled apricot mixture evenly over the dough in the pan.

Place a sheet of wax paper on a work surface and dust it lightly with flour. With lightly floured hands, pat the remaining dough into an 8-inch square about ¼ inch thick. Use the wax paper to transfer the dough to the pan and place it dough-side down over the apricot mixture. Remove the wax paper.

Bake until golden brown on top, 20 to 25 minutes. Let cool completely in the pan and then use the foil to lift it out of the pan and onto a cutting board. Cut into 16 squares.

To store: Transfer to an airtight container at room temperature for up to 3 days.

PIZZETTAS WITH BUTTERNUT SQUASH AND BABY BROCCOLINI

MAKES 2 MINI PIZZAS

A few smartly chosen convenience foods make these individual B1-packed pizzas a snap to prepare. Premade pizza dough is sold by the pound in many markets, including Trader Joe's. Frozen cubed butternut squash is preblanched, so it finishes cooking on the pizza. Mash the squash and chop the broccolini into small pieces to make a toddler-friendly veggie topping. Wrap any leftovers and refrigerate for up to 2 days.

Olive oil for brushing, plus 2 teaspoons
Cornmeal for dusting
½ pound whole-wheat pizza dough
1 garlic clove, smashed and then peeled
½ bunch baby broccolini, rinsed, ends trimmed, and roughly chopped
Sea salt
½ cup diced frozen butternut squash, thawed
½ cup shredded mozzarella cheese

Position a rack in the lowest part of the oven and preheat to 400°F. Lightly oil a baking sheet and dust it and a work surface with cornmeal.

Place the dough on the work surface and use a large sharp knife to cut it in half. Pat and stretch each piece into a 7-inch round and place on the prepared baking sheet. Set aside.

In a frying pan over medium heat, warm the 2 teaspoons olive oil. Add the garlic and cook just until fragrant, about 1 minute. Add the broccolini, sprinkle lightly with salt, and cook, stirring frequently, until bright green and coated with oil, about 2 minutes. Add 2 to 4 tablespoons water to the pan and cook the broccolini until soft, 3 to 4 minutes more. Drain the broccolini well and discard the garlic.

Place the squash in a small bowl and mash it with a fork.

Sprinkle each dough round with ¼ cup of the cheese and top with the squash and broccolini. Brush the edges of the dough lightly with olive oil.

Bake until the crust is browned and the cheese is melted and bubbling, 15 to 20 minutes. Let cool and then cut into pieces your baby can handle before serving.

WHAT'S HAPPENING?

Strong Bones. Congratulations to you and your 2-year-old! Your toddler is likely getting into more and more activities, such as jumping and throwing a ball. Even though her growth may have slowed down a bit relative to when she was younger, her bones are still growing and need nourishment to keep them strong and healthy. What should you feed her to support this? Magnesium-rich foods.

NUTRIENT OF THE MONTH: MAGNESIUM

As mentioned on page 74, magnesium is a really important mineral for baby's body. Although we usually think of calcium when we think of bone health, magnesium plays a crucial role in maintaining your baby's bone structure. Magnesium also aids in general tissue repair, nerve impulses, and muscle function, as well as moving stool through the intestine. Some baby-friendly options to boost magnesium levels include 1 ounce dry-roasted almonds (80 mg magnesium; puree to make your own nut butter), ½ cup boiled and pureed spinach (78 mg), 1 packet instant oatmeal (36 mg), ½ cup cooked black beans (60 mg), ½ cup cooked brown rice (42 mg), 3 ounces diced or shredded chicken breast (22 mg), or 1 cup diced avocado (44 mg). In addition to these foods, you can also try the following recipes to boost baby's magnesium intake.

QUINOA BURRITO BOWL

MAKES 1 SERVING

Use this as a template for a balanced, one-bowl lunch or dinner that gives baby a nice boost of magnesium from all of the ingredients. Pile your toddler's favorite cooked veggies, legumes, grains, and meat into a shallow dish and let him choose which bite to take first.

½ cup cooked quinoa or Herbed Brown Basmati Rice (page 154)
¼ cup cooked black beans
¼ to ½ cup diced cooked chicken
1 to 2 tablespoons shredded cheddar cheese
¼ ripe avocado, cut into small cubes
1 to 2 tablespoons diced red bell pepper

Spoon the quinoa into a wide shallow bowl and top with the beans, chicken, cheese, avocado, and bell pepper. Serve immediately.

SALMON STICKS

Making fresh versions of crispy, toddler-friendly frozen finger foods lets you control the quality of the ingredients. The secret to a flaky outer coating is panko bread crumbs, available in markets where Japanese ingredients are sold. Wild salmon is not only a great source of omega-3s, B and D vitamins, and protein; it packs a good dose of magnesium. Ask at the fish counter to have the bones and skin removed.

1 egg
1 teaspoon water
½ pound boned, skinned wild salmon fillet
Sea salt
1 cup panko bread crumbs
1 tablespoon olive oil

Preheat the oven to 425°F. Line a baking sheet with aluminum foil and lightly oil the foil.

Beat the egg lightly with the water to blend.

Cut the salmon across the short end of the fillet into ½-inch-wide strips. Sprinkle lightly with salt.

In a bowl, mix together the bread crumbs and olive oil. Dip the fish pieces in the egg and then in the crumbs, turning to coat evenly. Arrange them on the prepared baking sheet. Bake until the crumbs are golden brown and the fish is opaque in the center (cut one open to test), 10 to 12 minutes. Serve immediately.

To store: Wrap in foil and refrigerate for up to 1 day; reheat in a low oven.

TODDLER BANANA SPLIT

MAKES 1 SERVING

Happy birthday! This fun dessert is surprisingly full of magnesium—dark chocolate and bananas are both high in this important nutrient. Make a batch of this simple chocolate sauce and spoon it over ice cream and ripe bananas—add colorful sprinkles if you like—for a toddler-friendly party dessert to celebrate becoming 2 years old!

4 ounces dark chocolate, finely chopped
½ cup heavy cream
1 to 2 scoops vanilla ice cream or frozen yogurt
½ ripe banana, diced

Place the chocolate in a small bowl. In a small saucepan, heat the cream to a simmer. Remove from the heat and pour over the chocolate; let stand for 2 to 3 minutes, then whisk until smooth.

Scoop the ice cream into a bowl and top with the banana pieces and warm chocolate sauce. Serve immediately.

To store: Chocolate sauce can be made up to 1 week ahead. You'll need to reheat it gently, either in the microwave (microwave a few seconds at a time and stir in between) or in a heatproof bowl set over a pan of simmering water.

***

Congratulations! Your baby is turning 2 years old! What a wild ride it has been, and it will only get wilder. You now have a walking, talking small person, and thanks to you, he has started off his young life with a healthy relationship with nutritious foods. Not only have you exposed him to a variety of tastes but you have also ensured that he received all of the necessary nutrients to promote his healthy development. Moving on, in the next chapter, we will cover issues related to feeding baby in social situations.

Sample Menus for Ages 19 to 24 Months

These sample menus can give you some ideas for how to combine foods for baby. Feel free to mix and match to baby's preference.

ONE-DAY SAMPLE MENU—19 TO 24 MONTHS	
Breakfast	1 cooked egg ½ cup whole milk Medjool Date–Orange Salad (page 150) ¼ cup iron-fortified breakfast cereal
Snack	Almond Butter and Raspberry Jam Pinwheels (page 154)
Lunch	½ sandwich with canned tuna and ¼ mashed avocado 2 tablespoons black beans
Snack	½ cup yogurt mixed with ¼ cup iron-fortified cereal ½ cup whole milk
Dinner	2 ounces cooked ground turkey Herbed Brown Basmati Rice (page 154) ½ cup chopped, cooked carrots ½ cup whole milk

ONE-DAY SAMPLE MENU—19 TO 24 MONTHS	
Breakfast	Apricot-Oat Squares (page 164) ⅓ cup sliced banana ½ cup whole milk
Snack	4 or 5 crackers 2 tablespoons guacamole
Lunch	½ sandwich with 1 ounce sliced turkey, sliced tomato, lettuce Green Risotto (page 161)
Snack	¼ cup iron-fortified oats made with milk mixed with 1 tablespoon peanut butter
Dinner	Salmon Sticks (page 169) ½ cup cooked zucchini and yellow squash ½ cup whole milk

PART III

How to Help Your Baby Eat Well

7

Social Situations

While we tend to think of eating primarily as a strictly a biological process that we must engage in to sustain ourselves, there is, of course, a very strong social and psychological component to it. Humans congregate around food; they have throughout the evolution of our species. Even if you think about our eating behaviors now, most of the time people sit down with family members for a meal or go out with family and/or friends to a restaurant to eat.

Now that your baby has begun to master the fine art of eating, it's likely that some issues will come up related to eating out or eating with others. Let's tackle some common concerns and how you can address them.

WHAT TOOLS DO YOU NEED TO FEED BABY ON THE GO?

I have become a bit of a minimalist while traveling, largely because I found that the more I thought I needed when out of the house, the more I had to carry—and the more I could forget. If your baby is young and new to feeding, bring a soft spoon for eating out; but in a pinch, the plastic ones that most places offer will work just fine. Also, bring an old bib, possibly one that you are about to throw away anyway, so if it gets soggy you can just leave it behind rather than carrying it around all day. You can also use a cloth napkin as a bib (or even a paper one, as long as you watch that baby doesn't try to put it in his mouth).

Eating Out

I am a strong advocate for taking baby out to restaurants at a young age. I think it is important that parents still maintain a sense of adultness about their lives and find ways to include baby in it. So if you liked shopping and having lunch before baby was born, don't think you need to give that up or always get a babysitter. Baby can come along and be your lunch date!

But there are a few key things to keep in mind when eating out with baby. If you consider these and act accordingly, you can make the meal less stressful.

1. Go someplace family-friendly where you can make a quick exit. Don't go to lunch at noon when the rest of the world is on their lunch hour. Do an early or late lunch so you don't have to wait for a table. Also, if you have a stroller and baby will not be sitting in it, see if the restaurant has a special place where they want you to stash it. If baby is still an infant, it can be easier to prop the car seat in a booth next to you than to navigate a bulky stroller around a restaurant. And ask the person seating you for a place on the side of the room, so you don't have to bump into others if you have to get up with the baby.

2. Bring stuff for baby to do. Lots of restaurants have crayons and small things for toddlers and older kids to use but it is also a good idea to bring along some reinforcements, just in case. I suggest disposable reinforcements. You can bring some stickers, a few old crayons, and a mini tub of Play-Doh, and throw it all in the trash when you are done eating. Avoid bringing things that are valuable or expensive, as you don't want to worry about leaving something behind. Didn't bring anything fun for baby? No problem! You can also entertain your baby with stuff on the table. You may be surprised to know how fun sorting sugar packets can be for a 20-month-old!

3. Tell the staff what you need, right away. As soon as you arrive, let them know if you need a high chair or booster. Once you're seated, ask for a kid-friendly cup of water and extra napkins. It also can help if you tell the server right away what your baby will be eating, so she can place the order and baby's food can come out sooner than yours. If you brought baby's food, you can feed her while you are waiting for your food, and then let her play with stuff on the table while you eat.

4. Find your place. If you find a place that works well for you and baby to dine, keep going back. You might also want to befriend the waitstaff, in general but also to be able to ask for a broom to sweep up any mess baby

what to feed your baby & toddler

made on the floor. I make this offer all of the time, and not once have they ever let me actually sweep it up; it just is a nice way to let the waitstaff know that you know you made a mess. They get it, and they appreciate the gesture.

5. Ignore other people. I think for most parents, the anxiety about taking baby out to eat is the fear that she will act up and others will stare at you. Right? If that is how you feel, it is completely normal. None of us wants to draw unnecessary attention to ourselves, but you have to keep it in the proper context. People know that babies cry, throw things, and make noise. They should expect that possibility, within reason, when they go to a family-friendly place. So if you feel like you are getting icy stares from non-kid-toting people, just ignore them and tend to your child. Baby has every right to be a baby.

6. Don't leave just yet. If baby does start to fuss, don't feel you must leave the restaurant immediately. Maybe you can get up and go to the restroom and do a quick diaper check instead. Sometimes baby just needs a change of atmosphere. If you get up and leave at the first signs that baby wants to go, you are sending him the message that if he acts up in public he will get his way. So try to stick it out for a while. And if you do end up leaving, make sure to let baby know that it is because the meal is over, not because he was being bad.

KIDS' MENU? ─────────────────────────────────

You might be wondering what you should feed baby when eating out. Kids' portions are huge, so if you do order baby her own meal, be ready to bring most of it home. While some restaurants try to make their kids' menus more gourmet, most stick to the traditional kid fare (hot dogs, pizza, cheeseburgers, and so on), which is usually not very healthful. So a better option when dining out might be to order from the adult menu for baby. If you are ordering something that you could share with her, you can just ask the waitstaff for an extra plate. Sharing your meal is a good way for baby to try new things. Just make sure the texture and size are appropriate for her to handle.

When Baby Is Being Fed by Others: Day Care and Babysitters

While we may want to do it all, there will be times when baby will need to be fed while in the care of someone besides Mom or Dad. Here are some tips for making it a smooth transition.

1. Know your day care. Most day-care facilities are very accommodating to the requests of parents, especially when it comes to food. Inquire whether they have a policy about foods from home. Some prefer that you not bring food in glass containers (a safety issue, as they are breakable), so it is a good idea to ask before you invest in a set that you will use to transport home-prepared food for baby.

2. Let your caregiver know your concerns. Caregivers appreciate written directions. It is always easier to make someone happy if they tell you what will make them happy. If you want to know how much baby is eating, ask the caregiver to take notes, or leave the leftovers so you can see for yourself. If you don't need the details, that's fine too. Just tell your caregiver what you expect. Communication is key! Also, be clear about what you want your toddler to have in terms of snacks and sweet treats. This can be tricky when baby is in day care, where it can seem as if every day is someone's birthday.

3. Be flexible. If you have a certain menu that you want baby to follow, and Grandma is babysitting and decides to instead feed her something else (perhaps something that is on the not-so-healthy side), consider letting it go. Remember that once in a while it is fine for baby to eat outside the box (literally!). Also, be mindful that grandparents, in particular, don't always take your advice or recommendations seriously. So if your requests get ignored now and then, try not to sweat it. It probably isn't meant to dismiss your wishes, but many people just don't take dietary choices and healthy eating very seriously, unless there is an allergy involved. But if you find that baby is consistently being given foods that you don't want her to eat, do speak up and be firm about what you expect.

DON'T SWEAT THE SMALL STUFF ———————————

I remember the day my father-in-law dipped my 4-month-old daughter's pacifier into his ginger ale and stuck it into her mouth. If you'd seen my reaction, you would have thought he'd dipped it in acid! In hindsight, it was a completely innocent gesture; he was just trying to help because

what to feed your baby & toddler

she was teething, and back in the day, people did give sugar water to make baby feel better. (In fact, they still do. Many doctors recommend giving sugar water as a comfort for pain after circumcision—yikes!—or vaccines.) Ultimately, his act was also harmless, as my daughter is now 9 years old, and I don't think she even knows what ginger ale is! But at the time, I got very upset because I had made a very big point about how healthy eating would be a priority for her, and sugary soda wasn't on the list. Things like this are bound to happen, so unless they keep happening, try not to let them bother you.

PLAYDATES

Playdates can be a fun way for your baby to socialize and practice skills like sharing and having good manners. Often, playdates involve some snacks, and it can get awkward if you are trying to be mindful about being healthy and your host puts out a bunch of junk food. The best way to handle this situation is to avoid it by bringing a healthy snack to share with everyone. That way, you can be sure that there is something healthy available.

SOCIAL SUPPORT TO HELP FEED BABY WELL

In the United States, we don't really have a formal system of social support for new moms and dads. Most of us get advice from friends or family, and some join a mommy group, but you have to seek one out. Also, to get advice from your pediatrician, you must call or go to his or her office, and frankly, sometimes it can be a hassle. No house calls here! Things are quite different in other countries, though. For example, in Denmark, new families are offered home visits by a health visitor (a registered nurse with special training in child health), which take place regularly up until the child is about 12 months old. The health visitor follows the baby's growth and development and helps you with any concerns or questions you might have related to becoming a new mom, including feeding the baby. The visitor also sets you up with a group of four to six other moms who live close to you and who have all given birth around the same time. You meet up once a week (at home or in cafes) to discuss your babies' development, as well as any challenges you may be having. The health visitor is present at the first meeting with the new "mummy group" to introduce herself and talk about the benefits of taking part in a group as well as give tips on how to handle the new baby and answer any questions.

As a new mom, especially when it is your first child, you need some guidance and advice on how to get through all these new experiences, and for some who live far away from their family or friends, it is especially important to find a way to connect with others in the same situation. This is where the health visitor and the mummy groups come in handy. And the fact that it is a free service (paid through taxes) means everyone can take part in it if they want to. I wish we had something like this in the United States!

***

In this chapter, I've discussed some social situations that may arise when feeding baby and some ways you can handle them. In the next chapter, I will cover questions that often arise about allergies, picky eating, and some medical conditions that can affect baby's eating.

what to feed your baby & toddler

8

Picky Eating, Allergies & Other Medical Concerns

When toddlerhood strikes, babies become more willing to let you know how they really feel about things, and this includes their dislike for certain foods. You may find that the angel who once let you feed him mouthfuls of nutritious purees does not want to be fed like a baby anymore! Also, now that baby is getting more variety in his diet, he may not want to eat what you have prepared, and he may have started to develop preferences for certain foods.

What to Do When You Have a "Picky Eater"

If baby knows what he does and doesn't like, try to roll with it! Encourage him to be the boss, and give him some options, instead of you deciding the menu each day. But do be mindful that you don't want to become a short-order cook; there should be some structure to the meal. Also, just because baby suddenly stops eating a certain food doesn't mean it is gone from his diet forever. It may be that he wants a break from a certain taste. Remember, part of the reason we have variety in our diet is to ensure that we are getting enough of the necessary nutrients, vitamins, and minerals we need to stay healthy. So baby's balking at a food might actually be a subconscious way to let you know he is in need of nutrients that he can better obtain from something else (which is fine, as long as that something else isn't a brownie sundae!).

Here are some tips you can try when dealing with a picky eater.

1. Let baby choose the menu, to some extent. He likes to be the boss, so let him, within reason! Pick three healthy foods and let him choose which one he wants as a snack. Many parents reflexively ask the question "What

do you want to eat?" Try not to do that, because toddlers will always tell you the truth, and the truth is that they usually want a sweet treat—or junk foods, if they've been introduced to these out in the world!

2. Sneak it in. On pages 17 to 18, we talked about how fruits can mask the taste of veggies—this can work with your choosy toddler. Just getting the hint of the flavor, over time, can lead baby to find it less off-putting.

3. Get some help. If baby has older siblings, get them to help out. Showing a toddler how fun it is to eat healthy foods can sometimes be enough to get your little one to join in. If you don't have older kids, take advantage of when they are around (like at parties) and try new things then!

Dealing with picky eating can be frustrating for parents, but you want to promote positive feelings and attitudes about food. Don't "make" your little one eat her vegetables, and if she is crying about it or very upset, think about a different approach. You should reinforce that baby doesn't *have* to eat a certain food, but that you want her to try it because it is healthy and yummy. Little ones age 2 and younger really can't process the concept of health yet, so rationalizing with your child might not be possible until she is a little older. However, even at this early age, you want to be mindful of making sure your toddler learns the appropriate response to make when she doesn't like a food. Teach her to say "No, thank you" as opposed to making a face. Also, if she wants to spit something out, work on getting her to do so into a napkin.

IS THERE A LINK BETWEEN PICKY EATING AND EATING DISORDERS?

If your little one is particularly stubborn about food, you may wonder if she is destined for a life of food struggles. Picky eating is normal in toddlers. A food that's a favorite one moment is despised the next. As kids age and mature, most grow out of being picky eaters and become more accepting of new foods. However, for some kids, picky eating is severe and can be indicative of an actual eating disorder, such as avoidant/restrictive food intake disorder (ARFID), where a food is avoided due to taste, smell, appearance, or even past experience. The way we respond to our children's picky eating also plays an important role in helping them transition through the phase healthfully, says Alexis Conason, PsyD, a private-practice psychologist in New York City who specializes in disordered eating behaviors in adults. Bottom line: If you are worried that this is more than just normal picky eating, talk to your pediatrician.

Food Allergies

From 1997 to 2011, the prevalence of food allergies increased by a whopping 50 percent in children under the age of 18 years old. Today, nearly 8 percent of children under 18 are affected by food allergies, with an annual economic cost estimated at $25 billion. Although boys seem to be more affected than girls, food allergies don't discriminate based on age, race, or ethnicity.

Several groups of foods known to elicit allergic reactions (also known as *food allergens*) contribute to most food-related allergic reactions (about 95 percent of them). Chicken eggs, cow's milk, fish, peanuts, soy, tree nuts, and wheat are the top seven allergens most likely to induce an immune response in children. Not surprisingly, many of these foods are common in Western diets, and typically it's mandated that their presence be included on product labels. For years, it was believed that all potentially allergenic foods should not be introduced to children until they were at least 2 years old, and this is still commonly practiced today. It was also believed that infants at high risk of developing atopic diseases, like eczema and asthma, should avoid some of these allergens until they were even older.

Common Food Allergens and What You Need to Know

ALLERGEN	YOU SHOULD KNOW THIS . . .
Chicken eggs	Is usually outgrown by school age
Cow's milk	Is usually outgrown by school age
Fish	Doesn't typically disappear with age; not reduced by cooking
Peanuts	Is increasing in Western countries; can trigger more severe, life-threatening reactions; raw and roasted peanuts have similar potency
Soy	Is perceived as a significant problem, but not as well researched as peanut, milk, or egg allergens
Tree nuts	Can include almonds, Brazil nuts, cashews, hazelnuts, macadamia nuts, pecans, pistachios, and walnuts
Wheat	Is the cause of both allergic reactions and celiac disease, which have different symptoms

Although parents should be wary of potential allergic reactions (for good reason), there isn't much strong research to support delayed introduction of potentially allergenic foods. In fact, these outdated recommendations were based on very few studies with various limitations. Today, the American Academy of Pediatrics states that solid-food introduction should not be delayed past 6 months of life, and *any* type of solid food, regardless of allergenic potential, should be introduced to your infant (in a form baby can handle, of course).

HOW COMMON ARE FOOD ALLERGIES?

Approximately 8 percent of children have some sort of food allergy, which steadily decreases to 1 percent to 5 percent in adults (see the cow's milk and eggs entries on the facing page). However, such estimates are taken from a handful of studies (about ten), and the prevalence of food allergies in the studies varies quite a bit, so these results may not be quite accurate.

What about peanuts? The American Academy of Pediatrics' recommendations apply to them too! Contrary to popular belief, the research shows that introducing peanuts to your infant between 4 and 11 months is associated with a *decreased* risk of developing a peanut allergy. Just remember that you shouldn't introduce your baby to raw whole peanuts because they present a choking and inhalation hazard. Instead, you can introduce these in the form of peanut butter mixed into yogurt, peanut butter blended with banana and thinned with milk, or maybe even peanut soup. Also, if you suspect baby could have a peanut allergy because one of his parents or a sibling does, any introduction should be done under the supervision and advice of your pediatrician or allergist (see page 188).

Food allergies are often brought up in the news and in conversation, partly because of the health risk they pose and also because of how frequently they can occur. It is especially important to know which foods may cause allergic reactions, who is at greater risk of developing a food allergy, and how food allergens should be introduced to your baby. So let's take a closer look at the most common food allergens and then discuss how these foods should first be presented to babies who may or may not be at a higher risk of having a food allergy.

Cereal grains: Wheat, barley, and rye all have a variety of proteins that can cause allergic reactions (such as storage prolamins, alpha-amylase, trypsin inhibitors, and glycosylated peroxidase). Many people associate these cereal grains with celiac disease, which is an autoimmune response to gluten (found in wheat). It is important to distinguish this disease from allergic reactions to these cereal grains, which have a different set of symptoms. Both cereal allergies and celiac disease, however, should be treated similarly: avoid products that contain these cereal grains!

Cow's milk: The proteins that typically spark allergic reactions in cow's milk are casein, beta-lactoglobulin, and alpha-lactalbumin. Milk allergies generally occur in young children, who usually outgrow it by school age. Be careful, though; in more severe cases, serious reactions can occur with just a few drops. Most infants who develop an allergic reaction to cow's milk will also be intolerant of similar dairy foods, such as sheep's and goat's milk.

Eggs: Allergies to eggs are also more frequent in infants than in adults, and many children will outgrow this allergy by school age. Infants are typically intolerant of two proteins found in egg whites: ovomucoid and ovalbumin. The allergenic activity of eggs can sometimes be reduced by boiling to completely solidify the egg, though this won't reduce the reaction for all babies.

Fish: The vast majority of fish species produce a protein, parvalbumin, that can cause an allergic reaction. These reactions do not typically disappear with age, and they are not reduced by cooking the fish.

Fresh fruits and vegetables: We tend to think of fruits and vegetables as perfectly healthful and benign foods, but these are vast, diverse food categories, and some infants may develop an allergic reaction to some types. Thankfully, because different varieties have drastically different protein profiles, there is not a lot of overlap, and often an infant who is allergic to a single type of fruit or vegetable is fine with all the rest. Many of the allergic reactions to this food group are caused by certain birch pollens. This will often result in a more localized reaction in the mouth, termed *oral allergy syndrome*. Thankfully, the allergen can often be destroyed by cooking, though not the allergen found in celery. Some other fruits, such as kiwi, trigger reactions from proteins that are not pollens, which are more stable when heated and are not destroyed.

Peanut: I mentioned peanuts earlier, but there is a bit more to be said. Allergic responses to this allergen are apparently increasing in prevalence in Western countries, and peanuts are partially responsible for triggering more severe reactions that can even be life-threatening. Not only do roasted peanuts and raw peanuts have a similar potency, but there is no apparent difference in the varieties of peanuts with respect to the severity of an allergic reaction. The proteins that cause reactions are two different types of storage globulins and an albumin protein.

Seeds: Mustard seeds and sesame seeds are known to trigger allergic reactions, usually because of a form of the albumin protein that they produce. Though the prevalence of allergic reactions to seeds is lower than for other foods, it is important to keep them in mind when introducing new foods to your baby. The proteins that cause reactions are quite stable and will be just as potent if cooked or heated.

Shellfish and seafood: The muscles of many shellfish and other seafood contain the tropomyosin protein (or similar proteins), that will sometimes cause allergic reactions. Some of the seafood that may elicit reactions include lobster, crab, shrimp, squid, and abalone. These proteins are also stable when boiled, so cooking seafood will not help reduce allergic reactions.

Soy: Similar to peanuts, the storage globulin proteins in soy foods will cause allergic reactions, as will a certain pollen protein and another inactivated protein (a thiol protease). Soy allergies, even though often reported in the media as a significant problem, have not been nearly as well studied as the peanut, milk, or egg allergens.

Tree nuts: The many different tree nuts known to elicit allergic reactions include almonds, Brazil nuts, cashews, hazelnuts, macadamia nuts, pecans, pistachios, and walnuts. As with peanuts (a ground nut), tree nut allergies are a result of reactions to storage globulins and albumin as well as a few more obscure proteins specific to each type of nut.

So can kids really "grow out" of their allergies? For the most part, don't count on it. Although a significant portion of kids who initially have allergic reactions to cow's milk and eggs can eventually lose their allergies around the time they start school, this is not always the case. We don't know much about why some kids grow out of allergies while others do not.

what to feed your baby & toddler

DO GENETICALLY MODIFIED FOODS CAUSE ALLERGIES? —

Another more general category of foods that some families may worry about with respect to allergies is that of genetically modified foods, which we covered back on pages 43 to 44. One benefit of several genetically modified foods is that developers specifically delete the proteins that often trigger allergic reactions. In other genetically modified foods, developers may introduce a protein from one plant species into another to help it grow more efficiently or larger. There is limited concern that a genetically modified food with a "foreign" protein could have an affect in the field because currently none of the proteins being used are known to be allergens. So regardless of your family's view of genetically modified foods, know that there is not much to be concerned about with respect to allergies.

When to Introduce Potentially Allergenic Foods

Let's shift now to how recommendations for introducing novel foods to babies have changed, both for families who do not typically have a history of food allergies and for those who do.

Interestingly, more and more evidence shows that an *early* introduction to allergenic foods might actually *prevent* the development of allergies to these particular foods. This is worth repeating: Early exposure to potential allergens may protect your baby from developing allergies! This same body of research shows that delaying food introduction might contribute to the development of allergic reactions. So if your family does not have a history of allergies, you should start giving your baby a variety of foods, including those that are known to be allergenic, when you start solids.

How do these recommendations differ if there *is* a family history of allergies? Well, the answer depends on the century during which you asked. In the 1900s, health-care providers recommended delaying a baby's exposure to potential allergens, as they thought that this would prevent food allergies from developing in infants at "high risk"—that is, babies who have first-degree relatives with allergic conditions. Parents were careful not to expose high-risk kids to foods such as peanuts until they were 2 to 3 years old. However, this advice was based primarily on the opinions of experts rather than on evidence-based recommendations. In the 2000s, accumulated research showed that late exposure was actually *increasing* the likelihood that a child from a high-risk family would develop some sort of allergic reaction. Therefore, as noted earlier for peanuts (which I'll discuss in greater detail shortly), the recommendations have been revised to reflect the importance and potential benefit of early exposure to allergens.

So what should high-risk babies, or those with immediate family members who have some sort of allergy, be given—and when? Most allergenic foods (see the following peanuts paragraphs) may be given to high-risk babies starting at 4 to 6 months old, but only in liquid form. This means that you can give baby small quantities of cheese, yogurt, cow's milk protein formula (not whole milk, due to other nutrition factors unrelated to allergeneity), eggs, soy, wheat, tree nuts in a butter or paste form, and fish and shellfish and then carefully observe whether any allergic symptoms arise. It's important to try to feed your baby these allergenic foods only after other foods have been fed and tolerated. Babies are quite prone to developing an aversive association, and it may be more difficult to introduce many novel foods if the first foods your baby tries trigger an allergic reaction. And if you, your spouse, or one of your other children has a food allergy, you should definitely get your pediatrician's advice on how to proceed.

Here is some more advice that may seem obvious but is still worth noting. If your infant has an allergic reaction to any novel food or you think your baby has a food allergy, talk to your pediatrician or primary care doctor. He or she will know best how to move forward.

If anyone else in your family has allergies, does this actually increase your new baby's risk of developing an allergy? The answer is based on only a few studies, which essentially show a mild to moderate increased risk for your baby. As I already mentioned, exposing your baby to most allergens early rather than late may prevent him from ever developing an allergic reaction.

Peanuts

Research has consistently shown that if a sibling or parent has a peanut allergy, there is a significantly greater risk (about seven-fold greater) that your newborn will develop an allergic response to peanuts. If this is the case for your baby, you need to give her diet special consideration.

One particular study looked at the reliability of a peanut-allergy skin test in babies with siblings who have peanut allergies; this study also measured the willingness of families to introduce peanuts to their high-risk babies at home and their attitudes about the situation. The results were not too good. Namely, the study found that a peanut-allergy skin test in younger babies who have never been exposed to peanuts before is not reliable. In fact, most skin tests came up as negative, even for children who later developed a peanut allergy.

Moreover, parents strongly disliked giving their high-risk infant peanuts at home and were quite anxious before, during, and after.

So how should you proceed if your infant has a sibling or parent with a peanut allergy? If possible, give your child some sort of liquid peanut at the doctor's office. This controlled experiment with medical care at hand very likely will lower your anxiety and give you a more accurate test to determine whether your baby has a peanut allergy, and it *may* even prevent him from ever developing a peanut allergy. Of course, sometimes allergies are simply engrained in one's genetics and are unavoidable, but it can't hurt to try!

To summarize allergies in children, the overall prevalence is quite low, with a slightly increased risk if other family members already have some sort of allergy. *Early* exposure may prevent your child from ever developing an allergic reaction. Finally, if you are ever unsure about whether your child may have a food allergy, talk to your doctor. And if you are feeding your baby and think you observe an allergic reaction to the food, call your pediatrician right away, and if the baby shows any signs of difficulty breathing or swelling in the face or body, call 911 to get medical help immediately.

IS THERE A LINK BETWEEN CERTAIN FOODS AND AUTISM?

There have been lots of media stories about certain diets "curing" or reducing symptoms of autism in children. But is this real? Dr. Alycia Halladay, chief science officer of the Autism Science Foundation (and mom of two), says that the rate of autism is now at one in sixty-eight individuals and the prevalence has increased significantly over the last two decades. This obviously triggers concerns for parents about their newborn and what, if anything, they can do to influence whether or not their baby has autism. First, parents should know that autism originates prenatally and is highly genetic. Second, they should learn the early signs and symptoms that can be seen in babies as young as 6 months of age. Helpful information is at the CDC Learn the Signs Act Early website: www.cdc.gov/ncbddd/actearly. Early detection, diagnosis, and intervention can make a significant difference. Last, parents should know that formula feeding has *not* been linked to autism. The effects of breastfeeding are no different in those with autism than those without autism, but it is very common for infants with autism to have feeding issues. If this is a concern, ask your pediatrician. And there is no evidence that feeding a toddler a gluten-free/casein-free diet to potentially prevent autism has any effect.

Diet alone doesn't cause attention-deficit/hyperactivity disorder (ADHD), but studies suggest that certain food additives might affect symptoms in some children with ADHD. While super-strict diets (like the Feingold diet, which eliminates all processed foods and many fruits and veggies) have not been shown to work, many doctors support the idea that dietary changes could be beneficial.

There has been speculation that synthetic dyes, flavors, and preservatives found in many commercially prepared and junk foods might contribute to hyperactivity or other symptoms of ADHD. While most researchers have felt the examination done in this area isn't conclusive, a few new studies may be changing this. An analysis conducted at Columbia University and Harvard University found that removing artificial food coloring from the diets of children with ADHD would be about one-third to one-half as effective as treatment with methylphenidate (Ritalin). But only a minority of children are particularly vulnerable to the effects of artificial additives, and determining which children are susceptible is difficult, though not impossible.

Should you avoid artificial colorings in foods you feed baby, in case he has ADHD? It is up to you. I advise minimizing processed foods for kids under 2 years old as much as possible anyway, not for fear of exacerbating ADHD symptoms but because we want to start baby off eating wholesome foods loaded with *nutrition*, not dyes.

Infant Feeding Problems and Disorders

Sometimes a baby can develop a medical condition that makes eating difficult or, in some cases, even impossible for a while. A thorough discussion is beyond the scope of this book, but if your baby has a severe medical condition (such as one that calls for tube feeding), see the resources on pages 203 to 205. Here, I will talk about less-critical infant feeding problems and some infant feeding disorders.

Infant feeding disorders can be tricky to pinpoint, because sometimes the signs and symptoms are actually associated with another disorder. Feeding disorders may include difficulty with basic skills such as grasping food (in older kids; it is totally normal for a young baby to have trouble picking up little bits of food), holding liquids and foods in the mouth, sucking, and chewing. For example, a baby who can't pick up any kind of food and get it to his mouth or a baby who can't close her lips and keep food or liquids from falling out of her mouth may have a feeding issue.

Babies with swallowing disorders (termed *dysphagia*) can show a number of signs and symptoms; these vary from child to child, and diagnosis is based on the severity of the feeding issues. The following table lists common signs to look for. If your baby is showing any of these, you should talk to your pediatrician.

Signs and Symptoms That a Baby May Have a Feeding Disorder

Arching of the back and body while feeding
Chewing problems
Coughing or gagging during feeding times
Difficulty in coordinating breathing with eating and drinking
Difficulty with bottle and/or breastfeeding
Excessive drooling
Excessively long feeding times
Frequent spitting up or vomiting
Fussiness or lack of alertness while feeding
Increased nasal stuffiness during meals
Poor weight gain or growth
Recurring pneumonia or respiratory infections
Refusal of different textures of food
Refusal to eat and drink food and liquids

Babies who have feeding issues are at risk for dehydration, poor nutrition, and choking, so it is important to get help early if you think that your little one is struggling with feeding.

There are lots of medical conditions that can cause feeding disorders. Cerebral palsy, cleft lip or palate, autism, premature birth, low birth weight, respiratory problems, and gastrointestinal disorders are all associated with problematic feeding.

Reflux

A common medical condition that can affect feeding in babies is reflux. Up to 50 percent of newborns can have reflux, but it is sometimes misdiagnosed as colic, and many babies (and parents) suffer through the pains and crying until it is properly diagnosed.

Reflux is a condition in which the contents of the stomach flow back into the esophagus, causing pain. Signs can include vomiting, hiccups, arching back when eating, irritability, waking up a lot, and crying, crying, and crying. Most babies grow out of this by age 2, and the great news is that many parents report that symptoms often subside when they start introducing solids!

If your baby has reflux, your doctor may suggest starting solids a bit earlier than you would with a baby who doesn't have it. Some may advise you to try this before resorting to medication. When you do feed your baby who has reflux, there aren't any special guidelines or foods to try. How babies react to foods will differ, so if your baby seems to get uncomfortable and show signs of pain after trying one food, you should switch to another food that you've found won't cause a flare-up.

***

In closing, a baby is *the* most special gift one can receive. It's easy to get caught up in the chaos that a baby brings; sometimes you need to sit back and reflect on how special your baby is, and how special you are for all that you do for this small person. I hope that this book has helped you and your baby get off to a good start when it comes to eating, and that the information, tips, and recipes have made it easier and more fun. I also hope you can see how food can be used to help our littlest people have a healthy life from the very beginning.

References

Introduction

American Academy of Pediatrics. (2017) Infant food and feeding. www.aap.org/en-us/advocacy-and-policy/aap-health-initiatives/HALF-Implementation-Guide/Age-Specific-Content/pages/infant-food-and-feeding.aspx. Accessed May 23, 2017.

Avena, NM. (2015) *What to Eat When You're Pregnant: A Week-by-Week Guide to Support Your Health and Your Baby's Development.* Berkeley, CA: Ten Speed Press.

Bocarsly ME, Barson JR, Hauca JM, Hoebel BG, Leibowitz SF, Avena NM. (2012) Effects of perinatal exposure to palatable diets on body weight and sensitivity to drugs of abuse in rats. *Physiology and Behavior*, 107(4):568–575.

CDC. (2017) Childhood obesity facts. www.cdc.gov/healthyschools/obesity/facts.htm. Accessed May 23, 2017.

Karbaschi R, Zardooz H, Khodagholi F, Dargahi L, Salimi M, Rashidi F. (2017) Maternal high-fat diet intensifies the metabolic response to stress in male rat offspring. *Nutrition and Metabolism*, 14:20.

Kramer MS, Kakuma R. (2012) Optimal duration of exclusive breastfeeding. *Cochrane Database of Systematic Reviews*, 8(CD003517):1–139.

Nyaradi A, Li J, Hickling S, Foster J, Oddy WH. (2013) The role of nutrition in children's neurocognitive development, from pregnancy through childhood. *Frontiers in Human Neuroscience*, 7(97):1–16.

1—The Importance of Diet for Babies

Agarwal S, Reider C, Brooks JR, Fulgoni VL 3rd. (2015) Comparison of prevalence of inadequate nutrient intake based on body weight status of adults in the United States: an analysis of NHANES 2001–2008. *Journal of the American College of Nutrition*, 34(2):126–134.

Anzman-Frasca S, Savage JS, Marini ME, Fisher JO, Birch LL. (2012) Repeated exposure and associative conditioning promote preschool children's liking of vegetables. *Appetite*, 58(2):543–553.

Bale TL, Baram TZ, Brown AS, Goldstein JM, Insel TR, McCarthy MM, Nemeroff CB, Reyes TM, Simerly RB, Susser ES, Nestler EJ. (2010) Early-life programming and neurodevelopmental disorders. *Biological Psychiatry*, 68(4):314–319.

Bocarsly ME, Barson JR, Hauca JM, Hoebel BG, Leibowitz SF, Avena NM. (2012) Effects of perinatal exposure to palatable diets on body weight and sensitivity to drugs of abuse in rats. *Physiology and Behavior*, 107(4):568–575.

Capaldi-Phillips ED, Wadhera D. (2014) Associative conditioning can increase liking for and consumption of brussels sprouts in children aged 3 to 5 years. *Journal of the Academy of Nutrition and Dietetics*, 14(8):1236–1241.

Caulfield LE, Richard SA, Rivera JA, et al. (2006) Stunting, wasting, and micronutrient deficiency disorders. In: Jamison DT, Breman JG, Measham AR, et al., eds. *Disease Control Priorities in Developing Countries* (chapter 28). 2nd ed. Washington, DC: The International Bank for Reconstruction and Development / The World Bank and New York: Oxford University Press. www.ncbi.nlm.nih.gov/books/NBK11761.

Forestell CA, Mennella JA. (2007) Early determinants of fruit and vegetable acceptance. *Pediatrics*, 120:1247–1254.

Forestell CA, Mennella JA. (2012) More than just a pretty face: the relationship between infant's temperament, food acceptance and mothers' perceptions of their enjoyment of food. *Appetite*, 58:1136–1142.

Forrest KY, Stuhldreher WL. (2011) Prevalence and correlates of vitamin D deficiency in US adults. *Nutrition Research*, 31(1):48–54.

Fox MK, Pac S, Devaney B, Jankowski L. (2004) Feeding infants and toddler study: what foods are infants and toddlers eating? *Journal of the American Dietetic Association*, 104:S22–S30.

Galler JR, et al. (2012) Infant malnutrition is associated with persisting attention deficits in middle adulthood. *The Journal of Nutrition*, 142:788–794.

Galler JR, Koethe JR, Yolken RH. (2017) Neurodevelopment: the impact of nutrition and inflammation during adolescence in low-resource settings. *Pediatrics*, 139(Suppl 1):S72–S84.

Gerrish CJ, Mennella JA. (2001) Flavor variety enhances food acceptance in formula-fed infants. *American Journal of Clinical Nutrition*, 73(6):1080–1085.

Gillis L, Gillis A. (2005) Nutrient inadequacy in obese and non-obese youth. *Canadian Journal of Dietetic Practice and Research*, 66(4):237–242.

Havermans RC, Jansen A. (2007) Increasing children's liking of vegetables through flavour-flavour learning. *Appetite*, 48(2):259–262.

Jones AP, Friedman MI. (1982) Obesity and adipocyte abnormalities in off-spring of rats undernourished during pregnancy. *Science*, 215:1518–1519.

Kim SA, Moore LV, Galuska D., et al. (2014) Vital signs: fruit and vegetable intake among children—United States, 2003–2010. *MMWR Morbidity and Mortality Weekly Report (MMWR)*, 63:671–676.

Laus MF, Duarte Manhas Ferreira Vales L, Braga Costa TM, Sousa Almeida S. (2011) Early postnatal protein-calorie malnutrition and cognition: a review of human and animal studies. *International Journal of Environmental Research and Public Health*, 8:590–612.

Mameli C, Mazzantini S, Zuccotti GV. (2016) Nutrition in the first 1000 days: the origin of childhood obesity. *International Journal of Environmental Research and Public Health*, 13(9):pii:E383.

Mennella JA, Nicklaus S, Jagolino AL, Yourshaw LM. (2008) Variety is the spice of life: strategies for promoting fruit and vegetable acceptance during infancy. *Physiology and Behavior*, 94:29–38.

Mennella JA, Reed DR, Mathew PS, Roberts KM, Mansfield CJ. (2015) A spoonful of sugar helps the medicine go down: bitter masking by sucrose among children and adults. *Chemical Senses*, 40:17–25.

Piaget J. (1963). *The Origins of Intelligence in Children* (M. Cook, Trans.). New York: W. W. Norton & Company, Inc. (Original work published 1952).

Roseboom T, de Rooij S, Painter R. (2006) The Dutch famine and its long-term consequences for adult health. *Early Human Development*, 82:485–491.

U.S. Department of Health and Human Services and U.S. Department of Agriculture. *2015 – 2020 Dietary Guidelines for Americans*. 8th ed. health.gov/dietaryguidelines/2015/guidelines.

Wallace TC, McBurney M, Fulgoni VL. (2014) Multivitamin/mineral supplement contribution to micronutrient intakes in the United States, 2007–2010. *Journal of the American College of Nutrition*, 33(2):94–102.

2—Feeding Baby 101: Do's & Don'ts

Al-Salem AH. (2014) Nutrition and caloric requirements for infants and children. In: Al-Salem AH, *An Illustrated Guide to Pediatric Surgery*. Switzerland: Springer International Publishing.

American Academy of Pediatrics. (2017) Infant food and feeding. www.aap.org/en-us/advocacy-and-policy/aap-health-initiatives/HALF-Implementation-Guide/Age-Specific-Content/pages/infant-food-and-feeding.aspx. Accessed September 1, 2017.

American Academy of Pediatrics. (2017) Portions and serving sizes. www.healthychildren.org/English/healthy-living/nutrition/Pages/Portions-and-Serving-Sizes.aspx. Accessed September 14, 2017.

American Heart Association. (2017) CPR Anytime Infant. cpr.heart.org/AHAECC/CPRAndECC/Training/CPRAnytime/CPRAnytimeInfant/UCM_473170_CPR-Anytime-Infant.jsp. Accessed June 28, 2017.

Bawa AS, Anilakumar KR. (2013) Genetically modified foods: safety, risks and public concerns: a review. *Journal of Food Science and Technology*, 50(6):1035–1046.

Brown University. (2017) Pediatric Nutrition Handbook. med.brown.edu/pedisurg/Brown/Handbook/Nutrition.html. Accessed September 7, 2017.

Burke DM. (2004) GM food and crops: What went wrong in the UK? *EMBO Reports*, 5(5):432–436.

Celiac Disease Foundation. (2017) Non-celiac wheat sensitivity. celiac.org/celiac-disease/understanding-celiac-disease-2/non-celiac-gluten-sensitivity-2. Accessed June 28, 2017.

Christou P, Twyman RM. (2004) The potential of genetically enhanced plants to address food insecurity. *Nutrition Research Reviews*, 17(1):23–42.

Cushing AH, Samet JM, Lambert WE, et al. (1998) Breastfeeding reduces risk of respiratory illness in infants. *American Journal of Epidemiology*, 147(9):863–870.

Environmental Working Group (EWG). (2017). EWG's 2017 shopper's guide to pesticides in produce. www.ewg.org/foodnews/summary.php#.Wal7CtyR6M8. Accessed September 1, 2017.

Golden Rice Project. (2017) www.goldenrice.org. Accessed September 1, 2017.

Griffin IJ, Abrams SA. (2001) Iron and breastfeeding. *Pediatric Clinics of North America*, 48(2):401–413.

Herman E. (2005) Soybean allergenicity and suppression of the immuno-dominant allergen. *Crop Science*, 45:462–467.

Huh SY, Rifas-Shiman SL, Taveras EM, et al. (2011) Timing of solid food introduction and risk of obesity in preschool-aged children. *Pediatrics*, 127(3):e544–e551.

Johns Hopkins Medicine. (2017) Feeding guide for the first year. www.hopkinsmedicine.org/healthlibrary/conditions/pediatrics/feeding_guide_for_the_first_year_90,P02209. Accessed September 14, 2017.

Kalies H, Heinrich J, Borte N, et al. (2005) The effect of breastfeeding on weight gain in infants: results of a birth cohort study. *European Journal of Medical Research*, 10(1):36–42.

Karp H. (2013) *The Happiest Baby Guide to Great Sleep: Simple Solutions for Kids from Birth to 5 Years*. New York: William Morrow.

Kramer MS, Kakuma R. (2012) Optimal duration of exclusive breastfeeding. *Cochrane Database of Systematic Reviews*, 8(CD003517):1–139.

Li R, Dee D, Li CM, et al. (2014) Breastfeeding and risk of infections at 6 years. *Pediatrics*, 134(Suppl 1):S13–S20.

McKeon TA. (2003) Genetically modified crops for industrial products and processes and their effects on human health. *Trends in Food Science and Technology*, 14:229–241.

Montana WIC. (2017) Infant feeding guide. dphhs.mt.gov/Portals/85/publichealth/documents/WIC/Families/Infants%26Children/InfantFeeding Guide.pdf. Accessed September 14, 2017.

National Safety Council. (2017) Choking prevention and rescue tips. www.nsc.org/learn/safety-knowledge/Pages/safety-at-home-choking.aspx. Accessed June 28, 2017.

Nationwide Children's Hospital. (2017) Choking hazard safety. www.nation widechildrens.org/choking-hazard-safety. Accessed September 1, 2017.

Naylor AJ, Morrow A. (2001) Developmental readiness of normal full-term infants to progress from exclusive breastfeeding to the introduction of comple-mentary foods: reviews of the relevant literature concerning infant immuno-logic, gastrointestinal, oral motor and maternal reproductive and lactational development. Wellstart International and the LINKAGES Project/Academy for Educational Development. pdf.usaid.gov/pdf_docs/Pnacs461.pdf. Accessed September 7, 2017.

Owen CG, Martin RM, Whincup PH, et al. (2005) Effect of infant feeding on the risk of obesity across the life course: a quantitative review of published evidence. *Pediatrics*, 115(5):1367–1377.

Parikh NI, Hwang SJ, Ingelsson E., et al. (2009) Breastfeeding in infancy and adult cardiovascular disease risk factors. *American Journal of Medicine*, 122(7):656–663.

Pisacane A, De Vizia B, Valiante A, et al. (1995) Iron status in breast-fed infants. *Journal of Pediatrics*, 127(3):429–431.

Preboth M. (2005) AAP clinical report on infant methemoglobinemia. *American Family Physician*, 72(12):2558.

Rollins NC, Bhandari N, Hajeebhoy N, et al. (2016) Why invest, and what will it take to improve breastfeeding practices? *The Lancet*, 387(10017):491–504.

Vennemann MM, Bajanowski T, Brinkman B, et al. (2009) Does breastfeeding reduce the risk of sudden infant death syndrome? *Pediatrics*, 123(3):406–410.

Victora CG, Bahl R, Barros AJD, et al. (2016) Breastfeeding in the 21st century: epidemiology, mechanisms and lifelong effect. *The Lancet*, 387(10017):475–490.

WIC Works Resource System. (2017) Guidelines for feeding healthy infants. wicworks.fns.usda.gov/wicworks/WIC_Learning_Online/support/job_aids/guide.pdf. Accessed September 14, 2017.

World Health Organization. (2008) Persistent organic pollutants (POPs). www.who.int/ceh/capacity/POPs.pdf. Accessed August 29, 2017.

World Health Organization. (2011) Exclusive breastfeeding for six months best for babies everywhere. www.who.int/mediacentre/news/statements/2011/breastfeeding_20110115/en. Accessed August 29, 2017.

World Health Organization. (2017) Vitamin A deficiency. www.who.int/nutrition/topics/vad/en/. Accessed June 28, 2017.

UNICEF. (2017) WHO/UNAIDS/UNICEF infant feeding guidelines. www.unicef.org/nutrition/index_24811.html. Accessed September 1, 2017.

3—Key Nutrients Babies Need

Agnoli C, Grioni S, Krogh V, et al. (2016) Plasma riboflavin and vitamin B6, but not homocysteine, folate or vitamin B12, are inversely associated with breast cancer risk in the European Prospective Investigation into Cancer and Nutrition—Varese cohort. *Journal of Nutrition*, 146(6):1227–1234.

Allen RE, Myers AL. (2006) Nutrition in toddlers. *American Family Physician*, 74(9):1527–1532.

American Academy of Pediatrics. (2012) Breastfeeding and the use of human milk. *Pediatrics*, 129(3):e827.

Aschner JL, Aschner M. (2005) Nutritional aspects of manganese homeostasis. *Molecular Aspects of Medicine*. 26(4–5):353–362.

Bhatia J. (2006) Fluid and electrolyte management in the very low birth weight neonate. *Journal of Perinatology*, 26:s19–s21.

Black RE, Victora CG, Walker SP, et al. (2013) Maternal and child undernutrition and overweight in low-income and middle-income countries. *The Lancet*, 382(9890):427–451.

Boubred F, Herlenius E, Bartocci M, et al. (2015) Extremely preterm infants who are small for gestational age have a high risk of early hypophosphatemia and hypokalemia. *Acta Paediatrica*, 104(11):1077–1083.

Castiglioni S, Cazzaniga A, Albisetti W, Maier JAM. (2013) Magnesium and osteoporosis: current state of knowledge and future research directions. *Nutrients*, 5(8):3022–3033.

CDC. (2016) Vitamin K FAQs. www.cdc.gov/ncbddd/vitamink/faqs.html. Accessed June 28, 2017.

Covarrubias-Pinto A, Acuña AI, Beltrán FA, et al. (2015) Old things new view: ascorbic acid protects the brain in neurodegenerative disorders. *International Journal of Molecular Sciences*, 16(12):28194–28217.

Drake VJ, Angelo G, Delage B. (2017) Vitamin A. Oregon State University, Linus Pauling Institute, Micronutrient Information Center. lpi.oregonstate .edu/mic/vitamins/vitamin-A. Accessed June 28, 2017.

Ehrlich SD. (2013) Vitamin C (Ascorbic Acid). University of Maryland Medical Center. www.umm.edu/health/medical/altmed/supplement/vitamin-c-ascorbic-acid. Accessed June 28, 2017.

Ehrlich SD. (2013) Vitamin K. University of Maryland Medical Center. umm.edu/health/medical/altmed/supplement/vitamin-k. Accessed June 28, 2017.

Ehrlich SD. (2014) Calcium. University of Maryland Medical Center. www.umm.edu/health/medical/altmed/supplement/calcium. Accessed June 28, 2017.

Ehrlich SD. (2015) Vitamin B2 (Riboflavin). umm.edu/health/medical/altmed/supplement/vitamin-b2-riboflavin. Accessed June 28, 2017.

Gidding S, Dennison BA, Birch LL, et al. (2006) Dietary recommendations for children and adolescents: a guide for practitioners. *Pediatrics*, 117(2):544–559.

Green R. (2013) Cobalamin supplements for infants: a shot in the cradle? *American Journal of Clinical Nutrition*, 98:1149–1150.

Hamosh M. (1991) Institute of Medicine. Committee on Nutritional Status During Pregnancy and Lactation. *Nutrition During Lactation*, 157–158. Washington, DC: National Academies Press.

Hochholzer W, Berg DD, Giugliano RP. (2011) The facts behind niacin. *Therapeutic Advances in Cardiovascular Disease*, 5(5):227–240.

Hoffman JR, Falvo MJ. (2004) Protein: which is best? *Journal of Sports Science and Medicine*, 3(3):118–130.

Kennedy DO. (2016) B vitamins and the brain: mechanisms, dose and efficacy—a review. *Nutrients*, 8(2):68.

Kerling EH, Souther LM, Gajewski BJ, Sullivan DK, et al. (2016) Reducing iron deficiency in 18–36-months-old US children: is the solution less calcium? *Maternal and Child Health Journal*, 20:1798.

Kleinman RE, Greer FR. (2014) Complementary feeding. In: American Academy of Pediatrics Committee on Nutrition, *Pediatric Nutrition*, 7th ed. (chapter 6). Elk Grove Village, IL: American Academy of Pediatrics.

Mayo Clinic. (2013) Vitamin B12. www.mayoclinic.org/drugs-supplements-vitamin-b12/art-20363663. Accessed June 28, 2017.

Mayo Clinic. (2013) Zinc. www.mayoclinic.org/drugs-supplements-zinc/art-20366112. Accessed June 28, 2017.

Mazur-Bialy AI, Pochec E. (2016) Riboflavin reduces pro-inflammatory activation of adipocyte-macrophage co-culture. Potential application of vitamin B2 enrichment for attenuation of insulin resistance and metabolic syndrome development. *Molecules*, 21(12):1724.

National Academies of Science and Medicine. (2017) Dietary reference intakes. www.nationalacademies.org/hmd/activities/nutrition/summarydris/dri-tables.aspx. Accessed September 2, 2017.

National Institutes of Health, Office of Dietary Supplements. (2016) Folate: fact sheet for consumers. ods.od.nih.gov/factsheets/Folate-Consumer. Accessed June 28, 2017.

National Resources Defense Council. (2017). The smart seafood buying guide. www.nrdc.org/stories/smart-seafood-buying-guide. Accessed September 2, 2017.

Paoletti G, Bogen DL, Ritchey AK. (2014) Severe iron-deficiency anemia still an issue in toddlers. *Clinical Pediatrics*, 53(14):1352–1358.

Pirola I, Gandossi E, Agosti B, Delbarba A, Cappelli C. (2016) Selenium supplementation could restore euthyroidism in subclinical hypothyroid patients with autoimmune thyroiditis. *Endokrynologia Polska*, 67(6):567–571.

Ross AC, Caballero B, Cousins RJ, et al. (2014) *Modern Nutrition in Health and Disease*. 11th ed. Philadelphia: Wolters Kluwer Health/Lippincott Williams & Wilkins.

Schaafsma G. (2000) The protein digestibility-corrected amino acid score. *Journal of Nutrition*, 130(7):1865T–1867S.

Schleicher RL, Carroll M, Ford ES, Lacher DA. (2009) Serum vitamin C and the prevalence of vitamin C deficiency in the United States: 2003–2004 National Health and Nutrition Examination Survey. *The Journal of Nutrition*, 90(5):1252–1263.

Torsvik I, Ueland PM, Markestad T, Bjørke-Monsen AL. (2013) Cobalamin supplementation improves motor development and regurgitations in infants: results from a randomized intervention study. *American Journal of Clinical Nutrition*, 98:1233–1240.

Ventura M, Melo M, Carrilho F. (2017) Selenium and thyroid disease: From pathophysiology to treatment. *International Journal of Endocrinology*, e1297658.

Wagner CL, Greer FR, Section on Breastfeeding and Committee on Nutrition. (2008) Prevention of rickets and vitamin D deficiency in infants, children and adolescents. *Pediatrics*, 122(5):1142–1152.

Wang Y, Lin M, Gao X, et al. (2017) High dietary selenium intake is associated with less insulin resistance in the Newfoundland population. *PLoS One*, 12(4):e0174149.

Wessells KR, Singh GM, Brown KH. (2012) Estimating the global prevalence of inadequate zinc intake from national food balance sheets: effects of methodological assumptions. *PLoS One*, 7(11):e50565.

4—Starting Solids (6 to 12 Months)

Alvisi P, Brusa S, Alboresi S, et al. (2015) Recommendations on complementary feeding for healthy, full-term infants. *Italian Journal of Pediatrics*, 41:36.

American Academy of Pediatrics. (2017) Ages and stages. www.healthy children.org/english/ages-stages/baby/Pages/default.aspx. Accessed September 14, 2017.

American Academy of Pediatrics. (2017) Portions and serving sizes. www.healthychildren.org/English/healthy-living/nutrition/Pages/Portions-and-Serving-Sizes.aspx. Accessed September 14, 2017.

Black MM. (1998) Zinc deficiency and child development. *American Journal of Clinical Nutrition*, 68(2 suppl):464s–469s.

De Cosmi V, Scaglioni S, Agostini C. (2017) Early taste experiences and later food choices. *Nutrients*, 9(2):107.

Griffin IJ, Abrams SA. (2001) Iron and breastfeeding. *Pediatric Clinics of North America*, 48(2):401–413.

Johns Hopkins Medicine. (2017) Feeding guide for the first year. www.hopkinsmedicine.org/healthlibrary/conditions/pediatrics/feeding_guide_for_the_first_year_90,P02209. Accessed September 14, 2017.

Larson K, McLaughlin J, Stonehouse M, Young B, Haglund K. (2017) Introducing allergenic food into infants' diets: systematic review. *MCN, the American Journal of Maternal/Child Nursing*, 42(2):72–80.

Mahan LK, Escott-Stump S, Raymond JL, Krause MV. (2012) *Krause's Food and the Nutrition Care Process*. 13th ed. St. Louis, MO: Elsevier Health Sciences.

Montana WIC. (2017) Infant Feeding Guide. dphhs.mt.gov/Portals/85/publichealth/documents/WIC/Families/Infants%26Children/InfantFeeding Guide.pdf. Accessed September 14, 2017.

National Academies of Science and Medicine. (2017) Dietary reference intakes. www.nationalacademies.org/hmd/activities/nutrition/summarydris/dri-tables.aspx. Accessed September 2, 2017.

Preboth M. (2005) AAP clinical report on infant methemoglobinemia. *American Family Physician*, 72(12):2558.

Pisacane A, De Vizia B, Valiante A, Vaccaro F, Russo M, Grillo G, Giustardi A. (1995) Iron status in breast-fed infants. *Journal of Pediatrics*, 127(3):429–431.

WIC Works Resource System. (2017) Guidelines for feeding healthy infants. wicworks.fns.usda.gov/wicworks/WIC_Learning_Online/support/job_aids/guide.pdf. Accessed September 14, 2017.

5—Finger Foods (13 to 18 Months)

American Academy of Pediatrics. (1992) The use of whole cow's milk in infancy. *Pediatrics*, 89(6); pediatrics.aappublications.org/content/89/6/1105. Accessed September 15, 2017.

American Academy of Pediatrics. (2017) Portions and serving sizes. www.healthychildren.org/English/healthy-living/nutrition/Pages/Portions-and-Serving-Sizes.aspx. Accessed September 14, 2017.

Oliveira MAA, Osorio MM. (2005) Cow's milk consumption and iron efficiency anemia in children. *The Journal of Pediatrics*, 81(5). www.scielo.br/scielo.php?pid=S0021-75572005000600004&script=sci_arttext&tlng=en. Accessed September 14, 2017.

WIC Works Resource System. (2017) Guidelines for feeding healthy infants. wicworks.fns.usda.gov/wicworks/WIC_Learning_Online/support/job_aids/guide.pdf. Accessed September 14, 2017.

6—Bigger Bites (19 to 24 Months)

American Academy of Pediatrics. (2017) Portions and serving sizes. www.healthychildren.org/English/healthy-living/nutrition/Pages/Portions-and-Serving-Sizes.aspx. Accessed September 14, 2017.

WIC Works Resource System. (2017) Guidelines for Feeding Healthy Infants. wicworks.fns.usda.gov/wicworks/WIC_Learning_Online/support/job_aids/guide.pdf. Accessed September 14, 2017.

8—Picky Eating, Allergies & Other Medical Concerns

American Academy of Allergy, Asthma and Immunology. (2015) Introducing highly allergenic solid foods. www.aaaai.org/aaaai/media/medialibrary/pdf%20documents/libraries/preventing-allergies-15.pdf. Accessed September 15, 2017.

Begin P, Graham F, Killer K, et al. (2016) Introduction of peanuts in younger siblings of children with peanut allergy: a prospective, double-blinded assessment of risk, of diagnostic tests, and an analysis of patient preferences. *Allergy*, 71:1762–1771.

Feeding Clinic of Los Angeles. (2017) Feeding disorders. pediatricfeeding.com/reflux. Accessed September 14, 2017.

Fleischer DM, Sicherer S, Greenhawt M, et al. (2015) Consensus communication on early peanut introduction and the prevention of peanut allergy in high-risk infants. *Journal of Allergy and Clinical Immunology*, 136(2):258–261.

Green TD. (2014) Feeding allergenic foods to babies and pregnant or nursing moms. Kids with Food Allergies, a division of the Asthma and Allergy Foundation of America. community.kidswithfoodallergies.org/blog/feeding-allergenic-foods-to-babies-and-pregnant-or-nursing-moms. Accessed June 28, 2017.

Gupta RS, Walkner MM, Greenhawt M, et al. (2016) Food allergy sensitization and presentation in siblings of food allergic children. *Journal of Allergy and Clinical Immunology: In Practice*, 4:956–962.

Harvard Health Publications. (2009) Diet and attention deficit hyperactivity disorder. Harvard Mental Health Letters. www.health.harvard.edu/news letter_article/Diet-and-attention-deficit-hyperactivity-disorder. Accessed September 14, 2017.

Herman E. (2005) Soybean allergenicity and suppression of the immuno-dominant allergen. *Crop Science*, 45:462–467.

Hong X, Tsai HJ, Wang X. (2009) Genetics of food allergy. *Current Opinion in Pediatrics*, 21:770–776.

Institute of Food Science and Technology. (2015) What's a food allergy? www.ift.org/Knowledge-Center/Learn-About-Food-Science/Food-Facts/Whats-a-Food-Allergy.aspx. Accessed June 28, 2017.

Kanarek RB. (2011) Artificial food dyes and attention deficit hyperactivity disorder. *Nutrition Reviews*, 69:385–91.

Koplin JJ, Allen KJ, Gurrin LC, et al. (2013) The impact of family history of allergy on risk of food allergy: a population-based study of infants. *International Journal of Environmental Research and Public Health*, 10(11):5364–5377.

Larson K, McLaughlin J, Stonehouse M, Young B, Haglund K. (2017) Introducing allergenic food into infants' diets: systematic review. *MCN, the American Journal of Maternal/Child Nursing*, 42(2):72–80.

Liem JJ, Huq S, Kozyrskyj AL, Becker AB. (2008) Should younger siblings of peanut-allergic children be assessed by an allergist before being fed peanut? *Allergy, Asthma and Clinical Immunology*, 4:144–149.

Mermiri DT, Lappa T, Papadopoulou AL. (2017) Review suggests that the immunoregulatory and anti-inflammatory properties of allergenic foods can provoke oral tolerance if introduced early to infants' diets. *Acta Paediatrica*, 106:721–726.

what to feed your baby & toddler

Sicherer SH, Sampson HA, Eichenfield LF, Rotrosen D. (2017) The benefits of new guidelines to prevent peanut allergy. *Pediatrics*, 139 (6): pii: e2064293.

van Putten MC, Frewer LJ, Gilissen LJWJ, Gremmen B. (2006) Novel foods and food allergies: a review of the issues. *Trends in Food Science and Technology*, 17(6):289–299.

About the Author

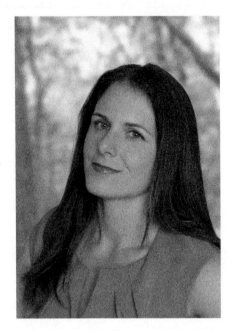

Nicole M. Avena, PhD, is a research neuroscientist and expert in the fields of nutrition, diet, and addiction. She received her doctorate in psychology and neuroscience from Princeton University in 2006. She then completed her postdoctoral fellowship at Rockefeller University in New York City.

Presently an assistant professor of neuroscience at Icahn School of Medicine at Mount Sinai in New York City and a visiting professor in psychology at Princeton University, she has published more than ninety scholarly journal articles on topics related to diet, nutrition, and overeating, and she frequently presents her research findings at scientific conferences and university symposia. Her research achievements have been honored with awards from several groups, including the New York Academy of Sciences, the American Psychological Association, and the National Institute on Drug Abuse. She has received research funding from prestigious sources, including the National Institutes of Health and the National Eating Disorders Association.

what to feed your baby & toddler

Dr. Avena's book *Why Diets Fail* reviews the research on food addiction and provides a way in which people can remove added sugars and carbohydrates from their diet. She has another best-selling book, *What to Eat When You're Pregnant*, that provides moms-to-be with nutritional advice on what to eat to ensure that they and their baby are healthy. She has also edited two academic books: *Hedonic Eating* and *Animal Models of Eating Disorders*.

A sought-after speaker, she has been lauded by her colleagues and the public for her ability to explain complex scientific principles and research findings to a lay audience. Dr. Avena makes public speaking appearances throughout the United States, Europe, and Asia to discuss her research and discoveries. She is regularly asked to speak to special-interest groups, industry groups, and schools. She appears often on *The Dr. Oz Show*, and she has also appeared on *The Doctors*, *Good Day New York*, *Home & Family*, and *The Better Show*, as well as many local news programs, including FOX5 San Diego, KTLA, WGN, and various New York stations. She has also been a guest on multiple radio programs and podcasts and has been filmed for several documentaries on the obesity epidemic. Her work has been featured in the *New York Times*, *National Geographic*, *Time*, *Bloomberg Businessweek*, *Shape*, *Men's Health*, *Details*, and many other periodicals. A member of the Penguin Random House Speakers Bureau, her TED-Ed talk, "How Sugar Affects the Brain," was ranked the second most watched (with more than five million views) and her video has been praised by educators and public health groups.

She also consults for many policy groups, pharmaceutical companies, and baby-food manufacturers and has a blog on *Psychology Today* called "Food Junkie," which explains relevant research findings in an accessible way. She also blogs for *Huffington Post*. You can follow her on social media at @drnicoleavena.

Dr. Avena lives in New Jersey with her husband, their two daughters, and their basset hound.

Index